Stretching
for **50+**

Stretching
for **50+**

A Customized Program
for Increasing Flexibility, Avoiding Injury
and Enjoying an Active Lifestyle

2ND EDITION

Dr. Karl Knopf

Published by:
Ulysses Press
P.O. Box 3440
Berkeley, CA 94703
www.ulyssespress.com

ISBN: 978-1-61243-671-5
Library of Congress Control Number: 2016957554

Printed in the United States
10 9 8 7 6 5 4 3

Acquisitions: Casie Vogel
Managing Editor: Claire Chun
Editors: Lily Chou, Shayna Keyles
Proofreader: Lauren Harrison
Indexer: Sayre van Young
Artwork: © 2017 Rapt Productions except © Robert Holmes pages 10, 11 (top), 12, 21, 47–48, 50, 52–54, 56–57, 59–60, 64, 66–67, 69–72, 75–79, 80 (main exercise), 87–88, 90–93, 96, 99–100, 103, 105–106, 111, 113, 117, 120, 122–23, 125–26, 129; © photobank.kiev.ua/shutterstock.com page 17; © kurhan/shutterstock.com cover image
Front cover design: what!design @ whatweb.com
Layout: Jack Flaherty
Models: Vivian Gunderson, Jack Holleman, Michael O'Meara, Phyllis Ritchie, Toni Silver

Contents

LOWER LEGS, FEET, & ANKLES

TOTAL BODY RELAXATION

PART ONE

Getting Started

Introduction

The secret to successful aging is to stay flexible in both your mind and body.

This book is designed for people who know that health and fitness are not achieved by luck but by staying active and doing as many good things for themselves as they can. The decisions we make daily, such as choosing to eat well and engage in regular physical activity, are the foundation of successful living. A simple rule of thumb for healthy aging is the 80-20 rule: Do healthy, positive things at least 80% of the time.

Most of us 50-plus folks were taught a number of outdated rules that could cause us more harm than good, including the old paradigm of "more is better," which leads many of us to overdo it. The intent of this book is to assist you to train smart, not hard.

In the '70s, fitness was all about aerobics; in the '90s, many of us started lifting weights. All this time, unfortunately, we neglected an important aspect of fitness: flexibility. Even now, we often fail to see how important flexibility is until we get hurt overdoing something, or our chiropractor or therapist tells us we have muscle imbalances (from poor posture, for example) that are manifesting themselves in chronic neck and lower back pain. To maintain a fit lifestyle, aim for 30 minutes of aerobic exercise five days a week, engage in strength training two to three times a week, and stretch daily.

I often see students who fail to see the importance of flexibility work until it is too late. They find themselves with hunched-over posture and a head that juts forward, which makes them feel and look older than their years. I find it interesting that folks will opt for plastic surgery, yet have poor posture that makes them look like Grandma Moses. Most poor postures can be improved with regular and sensible exercise done early on. I like the saying that most of the things that get worse with age can be positively influenced with proper exercise.

This book does not have hard and fast rules. The only rule in this book is to learn to listen to your body and heed what it says. The aim of this book is to teach you to turn inward and feel what is best for you. Throughout this book, you'll also find answers to the FAQs of stretching. No one knows your body better than you do! You are the captain of your ship, and everyone else is a member of your fitness crew. Never let anyone "should" on you!

A good relationship between your brain and muscular systems allows you to move with ease and comfort. Overly tight muscles can restrict a full range of motion, which can limit everything from your tennis serve to normal activities of daily living. Engaging in a systematic flexibility program can assist in undoing tight muscles that contribute to chronic pain and foster better functional posture. A daily dose of flexibility exercises will help you move with fluidity and grace.

According to the American Academy of Orthopedic Surgeons (AAOS), a stretching program can result in the following benefits:

- Decreased back pain

- Better circulation

- Improved joint mobility

- Efficient muscular function

- Enhanced posture

To get the most of these benefits, please keep the following concepts in mind as you navigate through the changes of the ages:

- Stretch what is tight and strengthen what is lax.

- Do unto your front as you do unto your back.

- Do unto the left as you do unto the right.

Remember that you hold the key to your wellness. Create the life you want. It is never too late to feel great! Too often as we age we think we are too old or too disabled to be active. Both are wrong! The key to happy aging is to change what you can and accept what you cannot. Try to remodel yourself daily; what you do today determines your tomorrows. With this mindset, you can grow well, not old!

Flexibility and Aging

The three S's that contribute to create an atmosphere for positive aging are strength, suppleness, and a sense of humor.

Have you ever woken up stiff and sore, or found that your shoelaces are a little farther away than they used to be, or that you need help getting your dress zipper pulled up? These are the little signs that your flexibility is decreasing.

Grab the skin on the back of your hand and hold it for a moment. Does it spring right back like it once did? As we age, we lose elasticity in our skin and connective tissue.

The reason for decreased flexibility is the result of many factors, such as muscle imbalances between agonist and antagonist muscles. A properly functioning neuromuscular system relies on the interdependence of muscles, tendons, as well bone alignment. An injury, misuse, or abuse of a muscle can disturb this delicate balance, setting up the cycle of inflammation, muscle spasms, and adhesions that cause adaptive shortening of muscles. Chronic malalignments, such as using one set of muscles while not balancing out the opposing muscle group, can lead to poor posture and chronic pain. One example would be a person who lifts weights and does chest exercises but does not balance that out by doing upper back exercises and chest stretches; this behavior would lead to a rounded shoulder appearance.

The key to aging well is to keep the proper balance of strength and flexibility in each joint region. The problem is that, too often, tight muscles get tighter and weak muscles get weaker due to sports or activities of daily living. This is why a daily dose of flexibility work is so critical. A good rule to follow is stretch what is tight and strengthen what is lax.

Aging results in increasing variability in terms of physiologic function. While no two people age in the exact same manner, most people can expect to lose elasticity in their skin and connective tissue with each passing decade. By the age of 60 or 70, we can expect to lose up to 50 percent of normal range of motion if we don't engage in a prudent flexibility routine.

Fit Tip: Most of the things that get worse with age can be positively influenced with proper exercise and stretching.

Benefits of Stretching

The most common flexibility limitations seen in the vintage body are osteoarthritis, effects from past injuries, and aftereffects of cancer treatments. If you have any of these, the good news is that poor flexibility can be restored! While it is best to engage in a prudent flexibility program before limited mobility becomes a chronic problem, it's never too late to begin.

A comprehensive stretching program will help you release muscle tension and soreness, as well as reduce the risk of injury. Just stretching a few minutes a day will assist in preventing soft tissue trauma such as muscle strains and ligament injuries.

Enhanced flexibility also fosters greater body awareness and a youthful posture, which leads to an improved connection between the mind and the body. A good relationship between your mind and your muscles allows you a better ability to move your joints within their natural ranges of motion. Keep in mind that the more efficient your movements are, the more easily daily tasks can be performed.

Overly tight muscles can restrict full motion in and around a joint. When muscles are flexible, joints can align themselves in the biomechanical manner in which they were designed. Improved flexibility results in improvements in everything else, from our ability to move, our posture, and even our ability to breathe more completely. Generally, poor flexibility and decreased joint range can be restored more easily if addressed early on, before it becomes a chronic problem. The longer the inflexibility exists, the more difficult it is to restore and the more likely it will become permanent.

It is easy to understand why flexibility training is short-changed. Unlike cardiovascular training that improves our heart function and assists in weight control, or strength training that improves our appearance, fosters bone density, and may even improve functional fitness, stretching just seems to be a perfunctory duty. While stretching may not reduce long-term health risks, it does improve posture and our quality of life. In fact, the AAOS recommends that people of all ages engage in a daily dose of flexibility exercises, which can include yoga, Pilates, and basic stretching.

A sensible flexibility program can benefit the following:

- Osteoarthritis
- Mobility impairments
- Effects of past injuries
- Aftereffects of cancer treatments
- Chronic pain syndrome
- Fibromyalgia

If you have any of these concerns and are looking for a holistic way to decrease pain and improve function, a daily bout of flexibility may be the solution. The longer the inflexibility exists, the more difficult it is to restore and the more likely it will become permanent. However, while it is best to engage in a prudent flexibility program before limited mobility becomes a chronic problem, it is never too late to begin.

What Is Flexibility?

Flexibility is the range of motion (ROM) around a joint and is specific to each joint—the more you are able to move effortlessly without pain or discomfort, the more flexible you are. Flexibility is influenced by many factors, two of which we have little control over: gender (women are generally more flexible than men are) and anatomy (the shape of our bones and how they form to make a joint). However, we can significantly improve our flexibility by stretching regularly, which this book will help you to do.

The types of physical activity that we participate in can make our muscles tight. Generally, the more muscular a person is, the more inflexible they are. When the same muscles are used over and over again, they become stiffer. We often overuse, misuse, and abuse our bodies in work or even play, which can lead to soft tissue injuries or even osteoarthritis. Joseph Pilates, the creator of Pilates, said, "The stronger the strong muscles get, the weaker the weak muscles become." This imbalance sets us up for injury, which is why stretching is so important. Overworking muscles can make us inflexible if we don't stretch, but being too sedentary may contribute to making us inflexible as well.

Why Is Flexibility Training Important?

Flexibility is considered an important aspect of a total-body fitness program. Unfortunately, many people neglect this part of their workout in favor of aerobics and strength training. If a person stretches, it is often just a quick series of bouncing toe touches or a few windmills. Unfortunately, as you will see, these types of stretches can cause more harm than good.

As we age, our ability to maintain independence through functional mobility is of utmost importance. Flexibility of our muscles and joints dictates our ability to perform our daily activities and avoid injury. Proper flexibility plays a significant part in how we stand, how we walk, and even how we maintain balance. Balance, in its various guises, is one of the keys to successful aging. This includes keeping your mind balanced with mental stimulation, keeping your center of gravity balanced so you don't fall, and keeping your body balanced by strengthening weak muscles and stretching tight muscles.

The *Guideline for the Promotion of Active Ageing at Primary Level*, published by South Africa's Department of Health, cites that lack of flexibility around a joint can cause functional limitations such as a shortened gait and rounded shoulders. Inflexibility can also make daily activities such as tying your shoes or zipping up a dress challenging. These incidences are small warning signs that your flexibility is decreasing and you need a consistent flexibility program.

In most joints, flexibility appears to peak around age 25 for males and somewhere between the ages of 25 and 30 for females. A preventive fitness routine that includes flexibility exercises begun in early adulthood can be the retirement plan for wellbeing later in life. While flexibility declines with age, studies have found that individuals who follow a consistent stretching program are able to delay and even reverse this degeneration. Most experts agree that loss of flexibility has less to do with aging and more to do with how we live and treat our bodies. You are what you do!

What Influences Muscle Flexibility?

A muscle is composed of elastic and non-elastic properties. The elastic properties are like springs that lengthen the muscle and return it to its pre-existing length. A sustained stretch allows the muscle and tendons to elongate gradually. Over time, biological changes occur in the muscle, allowing greater flexibility in the muscle-tendon unit.

Many factors influence flexibility, including the following.

Joint design. Ball-and-socket joints like the shoulder are more flexible than hinge joints like the knee.

Age. With age, most people undergo a loss of elasticity in the connective tissue and muscles.

Gender. Historically, females tend to be more flexible than men of similar age.

Physical Activity. People who engage in a comprehensive exercise program are more flexible than their sedentary counterparts. This may not be true in people who over-train and neglect a flexibility component of their training.

Temperature. An increase in body temperature or external temperature improves range of motion.

Pregnancy. During pregnancy, the pelvic region and ligaments become more relaxed.

Injury. Injury to an area can compromise the kinetic chain above and below the injury, which can have a negative effect of flexibility.

Specificity of Flexibility

Flexibility is specific to each joint. Unfortunately, this means that doing a stretch for the hamstrings will not keep the shoulder region loose. Another bit of discouraging news it that the benefits of stretching are short lived. This is why a commitment to a long-term stretching program needs to be adopted. A critical consideration is to make sure that the proper balance exists between antagonist and agonist muscles. If one muscle is too lax it can be just as bad as being too tight. The take-home message is that a balanced, slow, and steady stretching program needs to be done regularly.

Tune In to Your Body

As we get older, our bodies recover more slowly from various physical activities. Think of your body like a well-maintained vintage car that can often run just as well as a newer sports car but needs more TLC. The vintage car takes a little longer to warm up and needs to be tuned up more frequently, and so it is with our 50-plus bodies.

When you stretch, keep your movements controlled, maintain good posture, and really listen to your body—especially your neck, back, shoulders, and knees. When you are warming up, use this time to take inventory of your body and heed what it says. If you feel crunches in your joints, please don't ignore them. Listen for snaps, crackles, and pops—if they get louder or cause pain, see a doctor before they turn into real problems. Keeping our vintage car analogy in mind, it is always wiser and cheaper to do preventative maintenance than it is to do major repair work; thus, physical therapy is cheaper than surgery. Also, remember the two-hour rule: Two hours post-exercise, you should not feel worse than you did before you exercised. If you do, re-evaluate what you are doing.

Proper Posture

Proper posture is essential in preventing injury and muscle imbalances. This is how to stand with proper posture.

- Stand with your weight over the balls of your feet and heels.
- Tuck your tailbone between your legs as if you were resting on the edge of a barstool.

- Make the distance from your belly button and your chest as far apart as possible.

- Pull your belly button in.

- Place an imaginary apple under your chin.

From a side view, your ears, shoulders, and hips should be aligned. A mental picture that works for my students is to think of your body as a tube of toothpaste, with all the forces squeezing you in and upright.

When sitting, maintain proper posture by keeping your ears aligned over your shoulders and your shoulders aligned over your hips; the knees should be aligned over the ankles.

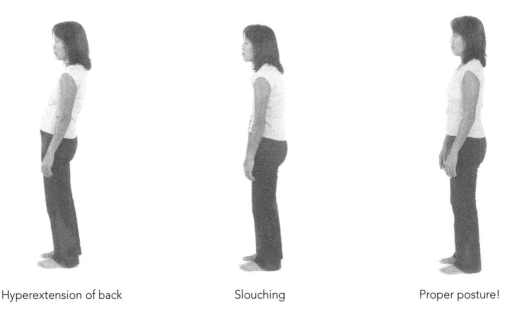

Hyperextension of back   Slouching   Proper posture!

Neck

The old expression "Don't stick your neck out" is excellent fitness advice. The neck is very fragile! Doing anything too fast or too hard can cause serious problems. Never "warm up" your neck by rolling your head around in fast circles—in fact, all quick neck movements are a bad idea. Avoid full neck circles because they strain supporting ligaments and can lead to pinched nerves. Other things to avoid include hyperflexion, when you force your chin to your chest, and hyperextension, when you arch your neck too far back. Neck extensions can also put pressure on the arteries of the neck, which can cause high blood pressure and compromise blood flow to the brain. Some women have had strokes while leaning back to get their hair washed at a salon, hence the term "beauty parlor" syndrome. The exercises in this book will show you safe and sane ways to increase the flexibility of your neck.

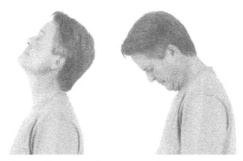

Hyperextension (left) or hyperflexion (right) puts undue pressure on the neck arteries.

Lower Back

Most of us will experience back pain at some time in our lives. It is critical to protect your back when you stretch. Keep your lower back stable at all times. All back exercises should be done in a slow and controlled manner, and if they increase in discomfort, *stop*. Never do stretches in which you bend forward and rotate at the same time: for example, windmill toe touches are a very bad idea. Also avoid bending backward at the waist, such as in yoga stretches that call for you to raise both hands over your head and look up. Quick, uncontrolled trunk twists are not a good idea, either, because torque generated by the twisting action strains the lower back. Be careful when doing fast or forced side bends, too. When sitting on the floor with your legs extended in front of you, be sure to keep your back flat when reaching forward.

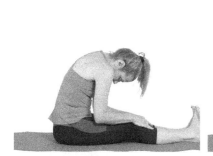

Bad: back is too rounded

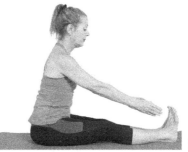

Better: back is flat but arms should be parallel to the ground

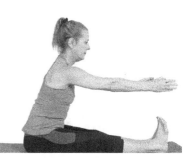

Best: proper form for reaching

Shoulders

Shoulder problems are an increasing concern for the over-50 fitness person. Be careful when you bring your arms above your head, and always control any movement that causes you to raise your arms above shoulder height. Relax your shoulders and don't shrug when you're doing arm exercises. Try your best to keep your shoulder blades pulled together when doing arm moves as well. If your shoulders are tight, don't arch your back to make up for your inflexibility.

Knees

The knees are designed to straighten and bend; any other movement is putting them at some level of risk. The knees and toes should always point in the same direction. Always remember: Keep your knees "soft" (that is, slightly bent) when stretching.

Avoid any movements that make your knees rotate or twist, and never twist your body while your feet are planted on the floor. Never straighten your knee so far that it hyperextends, or overly straightens the leg. Also avoid thigh stretches like the "hurdler's stretch," which cause your knees to bend too much. Forcing your knee to bend too far overstretches the ligaments of the knee and can make the knee joint unstable. Avoid deep knee bends, and make sure you don't squat any lower than the point at which your thighs are parallel to the floor. Always remember: Keep your knees "soft" (that is, slightly bent) when stretching. Lastly, don't allow the knee to extend past the toes.

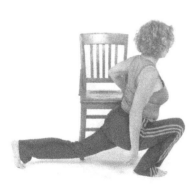

Incorrect: thigh is not parallel to floor and knee is extending beyond the toes

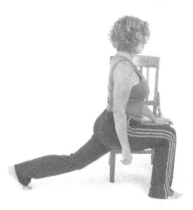

Correct: thigh is parallel to floor and knee is aligned with the ankle

Twelve Tips to Safe Stretching

1. When stretching, never twist your body quickly while your feet are planted on the floor.

2. Avoid stretches that hyperextend or lock your knee joint.

3. Avoid awkward thigh stretches like the "hurdler's stretch," which places too much torque on the knee area.

4. Avoid movements that force your knee to hyperflex, or bend too far, as seen in full squats. Hyperflexing overstretches the ligaments of the knee and can make the knee joint unstable in the long term.

5. Avoid neck exercises that take the joint to extremes or are done quickly

6. Always progress slowly and gently.

7. Select stretches that feel good to you. Not every stretch is best for you.

8. Two hours after a stretching session, you should not feel worse than when you started.

9. Make your flexibility session an integrated mind-body experience. Listen to your body and foster body wisdom. Turn your attention inward when you stretch, and try to exclude external distractions. Relax the mind, and many times, the muscles will follow.

10. If something hurts, stop immediately. Consult your physician for unusual or continuous pain.

11. Always warm up the body prior to stretching.

12. You are special, so treat yourself that way. Don't compete with or compare yourself to others.

How to Stretch

Structure follows function—what you do, you become!

We are what we do, so if you do stretches, you can become flexible.

Too often, active people focus on developing stronger muscles, improving aerobic capacity, or improving sport performance while neglecting the subtle aspects of fitness, such as flexibility. Exercising one particular muscle group without stretching it often causes that area to become less flexible and throws the body out of alignment.

Flexibility training is a planned and deliberate program done consistently with the aim of improving the functional mobility in or around a set of joints. It is an important element of a total-body fitness program. Still, improper stretching techniques can be harmful.

When stretching, always progress slowly and gently. You are unique, so don't compete with anyone else, or even yourself. Some days you will be pliable and some days you will be as stiff as a board—respect that fact, and keep it in mind when stretching. Whenever you are developing a stretching routine, always evaluate the benefits versus risk of each stretch. Not every stretch is right for everyone. Treat the selection of stretches in this book as a menu and pick only those that *feel* good to you. Two hours after stretching, you should not feel worse than when you started. If something hurts, stop immediately; consult your physician for unusual or continuous pain.

Be mindful of your movements. Move slowly between positions of lying down, sitting, or standing—don't overestimate your body's capacity to exercise. However, don't underestimate it either. Remember, your body is designed for movement, but let it adapt slowly and gradually.

What Are the Basic Types of Stretches?

There are two basic types of stretches. Ballistic, or bouncing, stretches are generally considered controversial. Research suggests that bouncing does not increase flexibility but can cause the stretched muscle to contract and shorten, which may induce strains or microtears of the muscle fibers. Static stretches, which are held for a longer period, are generally believed to be safer and more effective.

Remember to stretch opposing muscle groups equally in order to keep your body balanced. Our body is designed with opposing muscles. For example, you have a muscle that brings your hand to your mouth as well as an opposing muscle that takes it in the opposite direction. So if you do a muscle activity that brings your shoulders forward, do a stretch that opens the chest region up to prevent that from occurring. Stretch your tight muscles and strengthen your weak ones.

How Should I Breathe while Stretching?

Breathe fully while stretching. We often forget the importance that breathing has on health. Just think about how women use breathing to assist in delivering a baby!

Most of us take shallow breaths rather than deep, full breaths. Teach yourself to inhale slowly and deeply through your nose and exhale slowly through your lips. You will know if you are breathing correctly if your belly expands. Pattern yourself after the way a baby breathes. If you notice your ribs expanding, you are employing the wrong set of breathing muscles.

Breathing fully improves the quality of a stretch. An effective method for stretching a tight muscle is to inhale first and then exhale into the stretch. If you are tight in a certain muscle group, try reaching a comfortable distance, holding that position for a moment, taking in a deep breath, then exhaling and reaching a little farther. This is called the "hold/relax" method of stretching and relaxing.

How Long Should a Stretch Be Held?

Most experts from the American College of Sports Medicine (ACSM) suggest that maintaining a stretch for 30 seconds is ideal. After your muscles are warmed up, try to perform each stretch two to five times and gradually try to hold each stretch for 15 to 30 seconds. Start with what you are able to do. If all you can do is hold the stretch for 5 seconds, that is fine! If 30 seconds feels okay, progress to holding the stretch for 1 minute. Once a stretch feels completely comfortable, challenge your body to hold the stretch for longer or to reach farther.

Note that holding a stretch for 15 seconds provides better results than holding it for 5 seconds, and 30 seconds is better than 15 seconds. Some recent studies suggest that holding a stretch for 1 minute or more does not significantly improve the results of a stretching routine, but research has found no ill effects from prolonged stretches. No universal rule exists as to how long to hold a stretch—listen to your body! Aim for the ideal of 30 seconds to 1 minute, but be real. A 5- to 10-second stretch periodically throughout the day is better than no flexibility work. A little bit of any stretching is better than no stretching.

Never hold a stretch to the point of pain. Tweaking the position of the stretch to find the most comfortable position is A-OK. If you have not been stretching regularly for three months, hold the stretch for as long as it is comfortable, working your way from 5 seconds to 30 seconds. Note that you should not hold your breath while holding a stretch. The bottom line is that you should always listen to your body and avoid pain.

Why Warming Up Is Important

Think of your muscles as taffy. Imagine trying to stretch cold taffy: It would be difficult and snap. The same thing would happen for your muscles. Now imagine stretching hot taffy: It would be pliable and easy to stretch. Again, your muscles respond in a similar manner. If you try to stretch a cold muscle, you are at a greater risk of injury, so you should always increase the temperature of the muscles before stretching. A warm bath or light activity before you stretch is a good idea. Take time to warm up, and then stretch—your body will thank you later. Or, if you can only find time to stretch periodically throughout the day, pick times when your body is most pliable.

As you warm up, use that time to take inventory of your body. Listen to your body and foster body wisdom. Make your flexibility program an integrated mind-body experience. Turn your interests inward when you stretch. Reflect and relax. If your mind is uptight, it will be hard to relax your body. Some people enjoy listening to soft music while performing the stretch-and-relax portion of the program.

Safe, Functional Stretching

First, start with a warm-up. Active warm-up stretches are done slowly to lubricate the joint, increase circulation in the affected area, and make the muscle ready for movement. They should be performed in your pain-free range of motion. The active stretch is usually done as part of the thermal warm-up and as a post-exercise activity. If you have not been stretching regularly for three months, you should start out with 3 to 5 repetitions. If you find that too easy, you may want to shoot for 5 to 10 repetitions; if you are extremely flexible and have no joint disorders, try 10 to 15 repetitions.

Passive, or static, stretches are usually done after your body is warm, such as after a thermal warm-up or after an exercise session. Aim to hold static stretches for 15 to 30 seconds. The ACSM recommends that each stretch be done two to four times to elicit benefits. It is also okay to hold a stretch longer and do fewer reps.

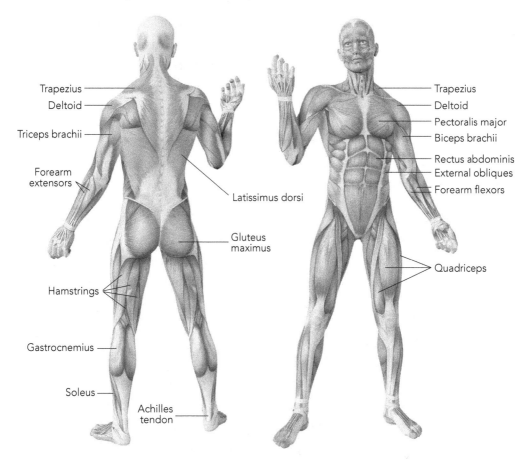

Trapezius
Deltoid
Triceps brachii
Forearm extensors
Latissimus dorsi
Gluteus maximus
Hamstrings
Gastrocnemius
Soleus
Achilles tendon

Trapezius
Deltoid
Pectoralis major
Biceps brachii
Rectus abdominis
External obliques
Forearm flexors
Quadriceps

Posterior view of muscles   Anterior view of muscles

While everyone is unique, the ACSM recommends stretching a minimum of two to three days a week. For best results, stretch five to seven days a week. It would be ideal if you could incorporate stretches in your daily routine, such as when in the shower or while watching TV. The more inflexible you are, the more often you should stretch.

As for which areas of the body need to be stretched, a total-body flexibility routine would be ideal. As you start out, focus on tight areas or problem areas. In most people, the chest, shoulders, backs of the legs, and lower back are often problematic. (In the Flexibility Self-Evaluations section starting on page 23, it is strongly advised to perform a basic flexibility assessment to help you ascertain where you are loose and tight.) As mentioned earlier, the human body is designed with opposing muscles, which are called agonist and antagonist muscles. A general rule of thumb is to stretch opposing muscle groups equally in order to keep your body balanced. The muscle illustration on page 17 will assist you in seeing the opposing muscle groups.

When stretching, think functional! Stretch those joints that you need in everyday life. For example, keep your shoulders flexible so that you can reach the cereal box easily. You don't have to be able to tie yourself into knots, but you want to be able to perform your daily activities without undue discomfort. Stay within your comfort zone, and don't ever force a move!

Remember, stretch what is tight, and strengthen what is lax. If, for example, you do an exercise that tightens your chest muscles, spend time stretching those chest muscles. As noted earlier, flexibility is specific to each joint. Try to stretch all the major joints of your body then focus on your particularly tight areas.

If you stretch correctly, you can avoid injury. It is safer and more effective to go slow; sustained stretches are superior to fast or bouncing stretches. If you ever become light headed while stretching, move slowly between positions of lying down, sitting, or standing. Don't overestimate your body's capacity to exercise. Let your body adapt slowly and gradually.

Be Your Own Motivation!

The more objections to stretching that you can come up with, the more you need to step up and be a leader in your health. The most common objections for not being involved in a flexibility program are not having enough time and being afraid of failure. However, we all have the same 24 hours to use in a day. The key to being a successful person is how you use those 24 hours. A stretching routine can be done in bed, in front of the TV, or even at work.

Goal Setting: Aim for Ideal, but Be Real

A flexibility plan without goals and objectives is much like a road trip without a map. While a trip without a plan might be enjoyable, it may not take you to your desired destination. If you want to get to where you want to go with regard to flexibility, you need to set goals.

Hopefully, you are currently motivated to start a flexibility habit. But, unfortunately, most people lose the excitement of staying engaged in a stretching program after just a short period. Most experts believe it takes 60 to 90 days to develop a habit, or 10,000 hours to be proficient in a new skill, so be patient with yourself as you develop your healthy stretching habit. Reaping the benefits of a stretching routine requires a long-term commitment. Setting lofty goals sounds impressive, yet it often leads to frustration. It is best to start by setting attainable short-term goals.

What you do today will determine how you feel tomorrow!
Nothing succeeds like success.

Methods to Foster Motivation

Starting a stretching program is easy, but maintaining it on a regular basis is difficult. A daily stretch program is drudgery for most people and agony for those of us who are inflexible. However, with time it should get easier. In this way, stretching is like flossing your teeth: You know it is good for you and easy to do, but it is much easier to neglect. The tips below will help you stay motivated and keep on track with your stretching goals.

Aim for ideal, but be real. An ideal goal might be, "I will do the basic stretch program from this book every day." A realistic goal would be, "I will do the Wake-Up Routine (page 30) three days a week." Not everyone will become a "Gumby" after reading this book. The purpose of this book is to encourage you to be the best you that *you* can be! Once you see progress, it becomes self-motivating.

Sneak a stretch in as a regular part of your daily routine. Do calf stretches while brushing your teeth, do a cross-leg stretch while sitting in a meeting, or do the zipper stretch while scratching your back.

Set up a support team. Surround yourself with supportive people. Even a million-dollar football player has a support team of coaches and cheerleaders.

Set up a reward system. Everybody enjoys rewards, so reward yourself! It is vital to establish a reward system as you continue to make progress. Set attainable objectives or milestones. Once you stretch daily for a month, treat yourself to a nice dessert. Once you can touch your hands together in the zipper stretch, buy yourself something nice.

Chart your progress. Some people like to keep a log of their progress to aid in staying motivated. Taking before and after photos is a visual way to see how much farther you can stretch than you could two months before.

Variety is the spice of life. Doing the same thing day after day is boring—even when we know it is good for us. If you change your routine periodically, you can keep stretching for a lifetime! Your hamstring muscle does not care if you stretch it while sitting in chair or while lying on the floor using a strap. The body does not care if you stretch during commercial breaks of your favorite TV show or at some trendy yoga studio—just make sure you stretch! And remember: "No pain, no gain" is insane, so do what's comfortable for you.

Dos and Don'ts of Stretching

DON'T stretch to the point of pain. Mild discomfort or tension is OK, but pain is not! Remember to breathe. Proper stretching should not cause pain.

DON'T engage in ballistic or sudden movements until fully limbered up.

DON'T rush and perform stretches incorrectly. You will only increase your risk of injury!

DON'T stretch if you have had a recent fracture, sprain, or strain, or suspect you have one.

DON'T overstretch a joint.

DON'T stretch if you suspect that you have osteoporosis or osteopenia. Speak with your doctor about what is best for you.

DON'T stretch if you have pain, discomfort, or an injury in a joint and around a muscle.

DON'T stretch if you have an infected or inflamed joint. (When in doubt, speak to your health professional.)

DON'T take joints to extremes, especially your neck or back.

DO warm up before stretching.

DO set realistic goals.

DO engage in static stretching.

DO change it up every now and then—don't get bored!

DO hold the stretch for 10 to 30 seconds.

DO design a flexibility program that focuses on tight muscles and incorporate the use of props to add variety to your program.

DO stretch daily, and enjoy!

Using Props

A flexibility routine can employ various tools like belts, balls, or a foam roller to enhance the experience. Props offer variety to your stretches. In this book, they are added to keep the programs exciting and increase flexibility. However, they are not necessary. If using props is a hassle and keeps you from doing the movements, then by all means, forget about them. Prop options range from the basic chair to foam rollers and straps.

The **chair** provides support in balance-challenging situations. Often a wall can be used for support and balance as well.

Foam **blocks** are often used in yoga to assist in maintaining a position. Blocks can serve as platforms for proper body alignment.

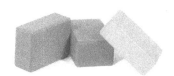

Foam blocks

A **pillow** can be used in the same fashion as a foam block; it can also be used to support your neck when lying down.

The **foam roller** can provide you with numerous exercises to improve posture, flexibility, and relaxation. Some rollers have knobs to stimulate circulation. They are a wonderful tool for releasing tension and adding diversity to your standard flexibility program.

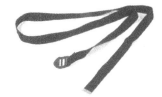

Strap with buckle

A **strap** allows you to reach the end stages of a stretch without compromising proper body mechanics. A rope or belt that does not elongate can be used instead of a strap. Other options include TRX suspension straps.

Resistance bands are typically made of latex and come in several shapes and intensities. There are basically two forms: flat and tubular. Some even come with handles attached. These elastic exercise bands are used in stretches where you move, such as the Torso Rotation (page 83), and to increase intensity.

A **stability ball** (also known as the Swiss or Pilates ball) is a popular stretching and relaxation tool. Some balls have knobs to stimulate circulation. Others have bumpy surfaces to promote sensory stimulation, while those with a hard, smooth surface are designed to provide trigger-point tension relief. They range in size from 45 to 75 centimeters.

Smaller, firm **therapy balls** also facilitate flexibility. The size, shape, and density of the ball you select should be determined by the goal of your session and, if applicable, the area of your body you aim to address. In general, tennis balls and other small firm balls (between 1 and 6 inches) with some give are good candidates for self-massage and muscle release.

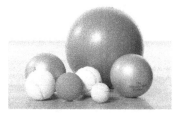

Therapy balls

Any device that facilitates your flexibility is acceptable. However, use your good judgment and always use caution when exercising.

It's important that you are comfortable doing stretches. When lying or kneeling on the floor, a mat provides cushioning.

Flexibility Self-Evaluations

Determining your current state of activity will provide you a baseline from which to start. Of course, it does not matter where you start but where you end up. The journey of many miles starts with the first step. Take a moment to assess your current level of activity. The following chart is a useful tool.

FITNESS LEVEL	ACTIVITY LEVEL
Athlete	Exercises, plays competitive sports, or has an active job
Currently Active	Exercises at least two times per week
Mildly Active	Weekend warrior; does yard or house work; exercises when time allows
Thinking about Exercise	Knows physical activity is good, but has health or time issues
On the Couch	Too busy to exercise; feels fit enough not to need regular exercise

Using the following pre-stretching assessments will help you better understand how flexible you are currently and provide you with an idea of which areas needs to be addressed. With this information in hand, you can design an effective stretching routine. Assess yourself periodically to see how your body is responding to your routine. Being honest with yourself is the first step to achieving your goals. Taking the time to evaluate your current level of flexibility will provide you with a point of reference to design a realistic flexibility plan and achieve your long-term goal. A simple assessment is if you find a stretch uncomfortable or tight, it may be an indication that you are in need of addressing that set of muscles. Most people who find a stretch uncomfortable will forgo working that area only to notice that region get tighter and more uncomfortable.

If you have health issues or concerns, consult your health provider for assistance and support. If you have had an injury, seek professional advice.

Side Posture Evaluation

Taking time to review your posture will give you an indication of how your tight muscles are manifesting themselves in a practical way. You can do this evaluation either standing or sitting.

Standing: Stand in front of a mirror and view yourself from the side. Your ears, shoulders, and hips should be aligned.

Seated: Sit normally in a chair and view yourself from the side. Your ears should be aligned over your shoulders, and your shoulders should be aligned over your hips.

Wall Posture Evaluation

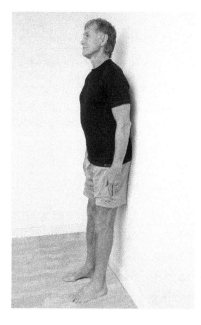 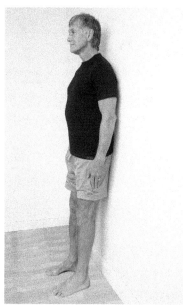 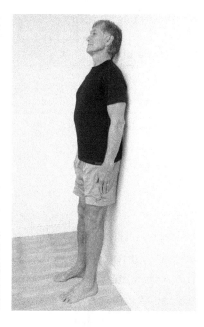

1. Stand with your heels 3 to 5 inches from a wall. Try to place your rear end against the wall.

2. If you are able to complete the first step, try to place your upper back against the wall.

3. If your rear and upper back can touch the wall, try to touch back of your head against the wall.

Posture Analysis

If the back of your head does not comfortably touch the wall, you probably spend a lot of time texting or leaning too far forward, which can lead to neck pain and headaches.

Intervention: Stretch the neck area gently and try the Head Tilt (page 43).

If you cannot get your upper back flat against the wall, your shoulder and chest region is too tight. You may notice that when you stand, your shoulders are hunched over. This rounded-shoulder posture can contribute to neck and shoulder pain and is often seen in people who sit at a computer or drive for long periods. This poor posture is common in people such as swimmers and weight lifters who do a lot of chest work.

Intervention: Strengthen upper back muscles, pectorals, and shoulder region.

If you have a significant arch in your lower back (also called a lordotic curve) when standing against the wall, it's possible that your hip flexor muscles at the tops of your thighs are overly tight. It is often found that people with tight hip flexors have a greater potential for lower back pain.

Intervention: Stretch out hip flexor muscles with Standing Hip Flexor (page 97) and hamstring stretches like the Sit & Reach (page 103).

Hamstring Evaluation: Sit & Reach

If you want to quantify your results, have someone use a ruler to measure the distance between your fingertips and your toes.

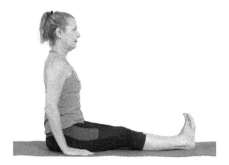

1. Sit on the floor with your feet straight out in front of you.

2. While keeping your back straight, attempt to touch your toes.

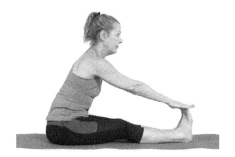

If you can touch your toes, that's good. If you can reach past your toes, that's fantastic! Keep up what you are doing. However, if you are like most people, you are not anywhere near touching your toes. If that's the case, this test is telling you it is time for a hamstring and lower back stretching intervention.

Intervention: Select several hamstring exercises, such as Figure 4 (page 108) or Straight-Leg Stretch (page 106).

Shoulder Girdle Evaluation: Zipper Stretch

If you want to quantify your results, you can have someone use a ruler to measure the distance between your fingertips.

1–2. Stand facing straight ahead. While standing, place your left hand, palm facing out, up your back as high as possible. Then reach your right hand, with your palm facing your body, over your right shoulder and down your back as far as possible. Repeat on the other side.

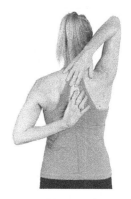

Can you touch your hands together? If so, great! If you can't touch your hands, you need to work on shoulder flexibility.

Intervention: Try shoulder stretches like The Zipper (page 62).

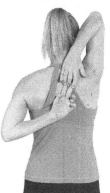

PART TWO

Specialized Programs

Programs Overview

Generally, as we get older, we lose flexibility. Many common chronic conditions cause us to "guard" or protect the joint, leading to further loss of mobility. Additionally, habitual overuse, either from work or from play, can hasten our loss of flexibility. This section provides you with some sample stretching routines for many common chronic conditions seen in the 50-plus group. It also includes stretching routines to accompany recreational pursuits older adults enjoy, as well as activities done day to day.

Feel free to do some or all of the suggested stretches. Try your best to stretch daily, whether you've been very active or have been sitting for a long time. It is better to do a little bit of anything than to do nothing at all. Just remember to listen to your body!

It was not that long ago that we were instructed to stretch before engaging in sports. Even today, if you attend a high school football game, you will see the players still performing bouncing stretches before a game, which is bad for the body whether you're 18 or 80 years of age. To prevent injury, the stretches in this book are all of a sustained nature.

It is ideal to warm up the muscles you plan to use with active stretches and a light jog or quick walk prior to doing any activity. Another good time to stretch is after a warm shower or bath, especially if you have osteoarthritis. Treat yourself like an expensive racehorse—no horse owner would ever allow her horse to go out on the track without being completely warmed up. So don't do anything, from shoveling snow to golfing, without warming up your body first. Note that warming up is *not* the same as stretching! Do a few minutes of light activity before ever attending to your daily chores or doing your favorite sport.

General Flexibility

The warm-up stretches I recommend in this program are good to do before any activity. However, the best results are achieved if the body is warm, thus a few minutes of light activity or a warm shower or bath will make the stretching session easier and more enjoyable. Start slowly and mindfully. The cool-down stretches, done after activity, will help your body release any tension or tightness you accumulated. In fact, some research suggests that post-activity is actually the best time to stretch to gain lasting results. If you're looking for variety, I've included a general flexibility program that incorporates props.

GENERAL FLEXIBILITY WARM-UP

Head Tilt, page 43

Tennis Watcher, page 44

Side Bend, page 81

Seated Knee to Chest, page 88

Standing Hip Flexor, page 97

Rear Calf Stretch, page 119

Gas Pedal, page 122

Ankle Roller, page 126

Shoulder Roll, page 57

Double Wood Chop, page 53

GENERAL FLEXIBILITY COOL-DOWN

Palm Tree, page 79

Sit & Reach, page 103

Seated Knee to Chest, page 88

Inner Thigh Stretch, page 101

Rear Calf Stretch with Strap, page 120

Self ROM, page 125

Finger Tap, page 76

Apple Picker, page 52

Elbow Touch, page 64

GENERAL FLEXIBILITY WITH PROPS

I, Y, & T, page 63

Mad Cat, page 128

Supine Hip Flexor, page 98

Hamstring/Hip Release, page 109

Ab Stretch, page 95

Torso Rotation, page 83

Side Bend with Band, page 82

Windmill on Roller, page 51

Elbow Touch against Wall, page 65

Novice

To get you started on the right foot, the next two programs are like the bunny slope in skiing, designed to see how your body responds to stretching. If you are flexible, you will find these programs very easy and sail through them. But for safety's sake, spend a week testing them out. If you find these stretches challenging, it is perfectly OK to stay at this level forever. It is also OK to modify the program to your skill set. Keep in mind there are no "musts" in this book. It is for your body, so personalizing the program for *you* is perfectly fine!

Always prepare the body with warm-up before any activity. Start slowly and mindfully. Once the body is warm, engage in gentle, active stretches.

STRETCHES NOVICE LEVEL 1

Head Tilt, page 43

Tennis Watcher, page 44

Seated Knee to Chest, page 88

Rear Calf Stretch, page 119

Gas Pedal, page 122

Shoulder Roll, page 57

STRETCHES NOVICE LEVEL 2

Sit & Reach, page 103

Seated Knee to Chest, page 88

Apple Picker, page 52

Elbow Touch, page 64

Picture Frame, page 61

Wake-Up Routine

Many of us with chronic pain or stiffness wake up tight in the morning. Many times, it is a good idea to take a few moments while warm and snuggly in bed to make note of which joints and muscles are clicking and clunking and limber out those creaks. Slowly move your body through a comfortable range of motion. Use your cat or dog as a model. Animals often stretch before they jump up and play. If dogs and cats do it, why don't humans do it? Sometimes getting up and taking a warm shower and then doing this easy routine back in bed is a good way to start the day, or even get ready to go to sleep.

BED STRETCHES

Knee Roll, page 85

Single Knee to Chest, page 89

Rock 'n' Roll, page 93

Double Knee to Chest, page 90

Gas Pedal, page 122

Pec Stretch, page 67

Chronic Conditions

Most physical therapists and exercise physiologists agree that most of the common chronic physical conditions can be positively influenced with sensible, regular exercise. Research has shown that everything from arthritis to multiple sclerosis can benefit from a gentle stretching program.

Many of the common conditions seen in older adults make the person stiffer, which can increase pain. Flexibility training can reduce muscle injury, decrease lower back pain, improve biomechanics, and reduce the stiffness of arthritis and other muscular-skeletal issues.

This section is designed to offer stretching routines for many common chronic conditions

Although all the stretching exercises in this book can be done by anyone, this section will address some common chronic conditions seen in mature adults.

Nothing you do should make you feel worse; if it does, cut back a bit and re-evaluate what you are doing. Don't be afraid to consult your health professional for a selection of stretches specific to your ailments.

Arthritis/Fibromyalgia

Stiffness is a common characteristic of osteoarthritis and fibromyalgia. Sensible stretching is of paramount importance in managing arthritis. Unfortunately, many people with arthritis complain of decreased flexibility, which results in a loss of range of motion. "Use it or lose it" really pertains to arthritis: If you don't move the joint, it will become stiffer and more painful, which can impair function. This is why a water exercise program designed specifically for people with arthritis would be an excellent complement to a safe and sane stretching program approved by your health professional.

When stretching with arthritis, follow these recommendations:

- always follow medical advice
- never over-exercise
- don't mask pain with medication
- never stretch a swollen or "hot" joint
- keep movement within the pain-free range of motion

Gentle stretching can be useful, as long as you stretch the parts you're using (stretching your legs will provide little or no benefit to the shoulder region). Lastly, remember the two-hour rule: If something hurts more than two hours after exercise, back off and do less next time.

STRETCHES FOR ARTHRITIS

Tennis Watcher, page 44

Seated Knee to Chest, page 88

Sit & Reach, page 103

Rear Calf Stretch, page 119

Ankle Circle, page 124

Gas Pedal, page 122

Seated Wrist Stretch, page 70

Finger Tap, page 76

Rotator Cuff, page 55

Shoulder Roll, page 57

Windmill on Roller, page 51

Hamstring Massage, page 110

Foot Massage, page 127

Frozen Shoulder

A frozen shoulder usually results from non-use of the shoulder because of a painful shoulder condition such as tendinitis or bursitis. If your arm is not used for a while, adhesions (tightness) may form on the sleeve-like structure that holds the ball-and-socket portion of your shoulder joint together. If the shoulder is not moved for two to three weeks, these adhesions will become very dense and strong and will result in a shoulder that cannot move freely—thus the term "frozen shoulder." If you have not been able to use your shoulder for a few months, consult a health care professional and follow a program under his or her supervision. Let pain be your guide: If stretching increases your pain, back off and follow the two-hour rule. It might be wise to warm up the joint with a heating pad prior to stretching and using ice after stretching. For other details on shoulder exercises, see *Heal Your Frozen Shoulder* (Ulysses Press, 2017).

STRETCHES FOR FROZEN SHOULDER

Shoulder Box, page 56

Shoulder Roll, page 57

Double Wood Chop, page 53

Hands behind Back, page 66

I, Y, & T, page 63

Prone Reverse Fly, page 58

Neck Massage, page 49

Hip Problems

Designed to support the load of our body, the hips are often called the workhorse of the body. Unfortunately, some people overuse them at their jobs, or in the weight room with heavy lifts. Sometimes, years of being overweight can put too much load on the joint and cause good hips to go bad. Consult your health professional for specific exercises for the hip joint. Avoid flexion past 90 degrees (allowing your knee to get too close to your chest) or crossing the midline of your body (when you swing your leg in front of or behind the other leg). For more details on hip exercises, see the *Healthy Hip Handbook* (Ulysses Press, 2010).

STRETCHES FOR HIP PROBLEMS

Sit & Reach, page 103

Inner Thigh Stretch, page 101

Standing Hip Flexor, page 97

Rear Calf Stretch, page 119

Gas Pedal, page 122

Hamstring/Hip Release, page 109

Quad Massage, page 116

Hamstring Massage, page 110

Side Bend with Band, page 82

Knee Problems

Chronic knee problems can be the result of poor anatomical design. If you are bowlegged or knock-kneed, you are at a mechanical disadvantage that can set you up for injury. Foot misalignments can also contribute to knee problems. In addition, injuries from sports such as football or soccer, or even too many step aerobics classes or badly executed stretches, can harm your knees. Your knee is an engineering marvel but can still break down if used incorrectly. Be careful to keep the knee in biomechanical alignment: Your knees and toes should always point in the same direction, and you should never over-bend your knees or over-straighten your legs.

STRETCHES FOR KNEE PROBLEMS

Sit & Reach, page 103

Straight-Leg Stretch, page 106

Standing Hip Flexor, page 97

Rear Calf Stretch, page 119

Rear Calf Stretch with Strap, page 120

Hamstring Massage, page 110

Quad Massage, page 116

Inner Thigh Massage, page 102

Side Bend with Band, page 82

Lower Back Pain

Lower back pain is caused by a variety of sources, including weak abdominals, tight hamstrings and quadriceps, improper body mechanics, poor posture, overuse, facet and joint problems, and herniated discs. Many arm movements affect the lower back, and activities such as overhead reaching affect the lumbar lordosis. Back problems should be diagnosed by a health care professional. A healthy back program includes exercises that strengthen the abdominals and stretch the hamstrings and lower back muscles. For people with back problems, learning about and performing the good neutral spine technique is very important (see Proper Posture on page 9). All exercises should be done from this stance unless otherwise instructed by your health professional.

STRETCHES FOR LOWER BACK PAIN

Single Knee to Chest, page 89

Double Knee to Chest, page 90

Sit & Reach, page 103

Mad Cat, page 128

Standing Hip Flexor, page 97

Piriformis Stretch, page 92

Windmill on Roller, page 51

Hamstring Massage, page 110

Double-Leg Stretch, page 111

Repetitive Wrist Strain

Repetitive injuries are caused from—just as they sound—doing any detailed task repeatedly without taking a break. The pathology that causes the problem is complex and needs to be explained by your doctor. It is interesting to note that carpal tunnel wrist syndrome really increased when computers became popular.

STRETCHES FOR REPETITIVE WRIST STRAIN

Seated Wrist Stretch, page 70

Standing Wrist Stretch, page 71

V-W Stretch, page 78

Band Roll-Up, page 74

Inward/Outward Wrist Stretch, page 69

Forearm Massage, page 73

Recreational Pursuits

This series is designed to prevent possible injuries, rehabilitate existing injuries, and balance out the negative results of one-sided activities, such as golf and tennis. For more specific information on sports conditioning, check out *Total Sports Conditioning for Athletes 50+* (Ulysses Press, 2008).

Biking/Cycling

Most people would assume that biking is a lower body activity, but think of your posture as you're on the bike. Your body is rounded over the handlebars, with much of your weight resting on your wrists and hands. Start out with an easy warm-up ride. If you're very inflexible, get off the bike and stretch. Otherwise, stretch after your ride and ice sore joints if necessary. If you can, have your bike professionally adjusted to fit you.

STRETCHES FOR BIKING/CYCLING

Single Knee to Chest, page 89

Standing Quad Stretch, page 112

Double Knee to Chest, page 90

Kneeling Hip Flexor, page 96

Piriformis Stretch, page 92

Figure 4, page 108

Rear Calf Stretch, page 119

Gas Pedal, page 122

Ankle Circle, page 124

I, Y, & T, page 63

Torso Relax, page 84

Hamstring/Hip Release, page 109

Quad Massage, page 116

Foot Massage, page 127

Bowling

Many people don't think bowling is a sport, yet it can be very hard on the hips, knees, shoulders, and back. One problem that bowling presents is that it is one-sided, and you are asked to throw a heavy ball with full force. All this can lead to injuries. Practice with a few easy rolls before going full strength.

STRETCHES FOR BOWLING

Sit & Reach, page 103

Standing Hip Flexor, page 97

Gas Pedal, page 122

Heel Raise/Heel Drop, page 123

Seated Wrist Stretch, page 70

Inward/Outward Wrist Stretch, page 69

Finger Tap, page 76

Finger Spreader, page 77

Shoulder Box, page 56

Head Tilt, page 43

Tennis Watcher, page 44

Side Bend, page 81

Seated Knee to Chest, page 88

Twister, page 80

Windmill on Roller, page 51

Drop-Off Stretch, page 121

Forearm Massage, page 73

Canoeing, Kayaking, or Stand-Up Paddle Boarding

Stand-up paddle boarding (SUP) and paddling sports like canoeing and kayaking are primarily upper body tasks, so pay attention to not getting overly tight through the chest region. Perform a light walk or jog beforehand. If you tend to use only one side to stroke, try to switch sides in order to balance out your muscle use.

Twister, page 80

Windmill on Roller, page 51

Tennis Watcher, page 44

Neck Massage, page 49

Pec Stretch, page 67

I, Y, & T, page 63

The Zipper, page 62

Standing Quad Stretch, page 112

Picture Frame, page 61

Golf

Many people say they play golf, yet I am still waiting to speak to someone who "plays" golf. Most people actually *compete* at golf, and often make an enjoyable pastime a stress-laden event. Golf is tough on the body and hard on the knees, hips, and especially the lower back. One problem with golf is that it is asymmetrical, meaning only one side of the body gets used repeatedly. The other issue is that the worse at golf you are, the harder it is on your body due to more repetition and bad form.

Walk for a few minutes before the match starts; walk the course, if possible. Don't always pull your clubs with the same arm. Similarly, try taking an equal number of swings to the left and right to even out all the one-sided swings you'll be executing in the game. Try to stay as balanced to the left as you are to the right. And, finally, avoid the food and drink at the 19th hole!

STRETCHES FOR GOLF

Turtle, page 46

Finger Spreader, page 77

Head Tilt, page 43

Shoulder Roll, page 57

Side Bend, page 81

Hands behind Back, page 66

Palm Tree, page 79

The Zipper, page 62

Double Knee to Chest, page 90

Elbow Touch, page 64

Rear Calf Stretch, page 119

Windmill on Roller, page 51

Standing Wrist Stretch, page 71

Prone Reverse Fly, page 58

Inward/Outward Wrist Stretch, page 69

Neck Massage, page 49

Skiing/Snowboarding

Skiing can be an explosive sport that asks you to perform hard for short spurts, stand around for a while in line, and then exert at full force again. With skiing, you have to contend with the cold at high altitudes, and our 50-plus tendons and ligaments often gel up when left alone in the cold. Skiing is a total-body sport, and can be hard on shoulders, knees, and tendons. Always warm up and stop when you are fatigued. Listen to your body. Don't over-ski your ability or fitness level. Ski a couple of bunny slopes before you start the day, and finish with a stretch after a warm shower.

STRETCHES FOR SKIING

Skyscraper, page 45

Palm Tree, page 79

Side Bend, page 81

Sit & Reach, page 103

Standing Quad Stretch, page 112

Standing Hip Flexor, page 97

Rear Calf Stretch, page 119

Ankle Circle, page 124

Seated Wrist Stretch, page 70

Finger Spreader, page 77

Double Wood Chop, page 53

Choker, page 60

Picture Frame, page 61

Over the Top, page 59

Kneeling Hip Flexor, page 96

Inner Thigh Massage, page 102

Hamstring Massage, page 110

Foot Massage, page 127

Swimming

Water exercise is gentle on the body and everybody should do it. But swimming is not as kind. Over time, swimming laps can contribute to shoulder problems, and breathing to one side repeatedly can aggravate lower back problems. A few gentle laps to warm up is always a good idea. Stretch after your laps. It would be wise to have your swim skills analyzed if you swim a lot.

STRETCHES FOR SWIMMING

Gas Pedal, page 122

Shoulder Roll, page 57

Double Wood Chop, page 53

Choker, page 60

Over the Top, page 59

Pec Stretch, page 67

Windmill on Roller, page 51

Neck Massage, page 49

Prone Reverse Fly, page 58

I, Y, & T, page 63

Torso Relax, page 84

Tennis

Tennis is a fun sport, but it often takes a significant toll on the body. The knees take a pounding and the shoulders are asked to perform some difficult moves. The load placed on the spine, not to mention the cardiovascular system, is tremendous. The fact that it is mostly an asymmetrical game (meaning it is done mostly on one side of the body) sets you up for misalignments.

Stretching is very important if you are a tennis player. Take a few minutes to walk around the court then gently hit the ball back and forth to lubricate the affected joints. Once you're warmed up, take a few moments to stretch before the game starts. Stretch between sets and after the game as well.

STRETCHES FOR TENNIS

Double Knee to Chest, page 90

Piriformis Stretch, page 92

The Butterfly, page 99

Inner Thigh Stretch, page 101

Rear Calf Stretch, page 119

Drop-Off Stretch, page 121

V Stretch, page 105

Ankle Circle, page 124

Picture Frame, page 61

Pec Stretch, page 67

Rotator Cuff, page 55

Windmill on Roller, page 51

Side Bend with Band, page 82

Kneeling Hip Flexor, page 96

Inner Thigh Massage, page 102

Standing Quad Stretch, page 112

Foot Massage, page 127

Walking/Jogging

Jogging, running, and walking are primarily lower body activities. To incorporate a stretching routine into your regular activities, start out at a slower pace than you usually do. Once you feel warmed up, stop and stretch your hips, legs, knees, and ankles. Don't forget to stretch your chest and shoulders, because often your upper body becomes hunched over. After your exercise, take time to stretch some more.

STRETCHES FOR WALKING/JOGGING

Double Knee to Chest, page 90

Standing Hip Flexor, page 97

Rear Calf Stretch, page 119

Gas Pedal, page 122

Ankle Circle, page 124

Windmill on Roller, page 51

Side Bend with Band, page 82

Kneeling Hip Flexor, page 96

Quad Massage, page 116

Hamstring Massage, page 110

Inner Thigh Massage, page 102

Foot Massage, page 127

Daily Activities

The following are some simple stretching routines for daily activities that seem innocuous enough but can cause problems when performed abruptly or for too long.

Gardening

Gardening sounds like fun to some and work to others. If you are not fit to bend, squat, or lift, perhaps window box gardening may be a better option. Warm up the body before you start gardening. If it is spring planting season and you have been sedentary all winter, use caution and don't overdo it.

STRETCHES FOR GARDENING

Tennis Watcher, page 44

Side Bend, page 81

Twister, page 80

Standing Hip Flexor, page 97

Rear Calf Stretch, page 119

Finger Tap, page 76

Apple Picker, page 52

Double Wood Chop, page 53

Mad Cat, page 128

Housecleaning/Lifting

Doing housework can be strenuous physical activity and should be performed with caution because it is very easy to strain muscles. Areas of special concern should be the lower back and knees. Walk around for a few minutes before doing chores and then stretch afterward. Protect your back and ask for help when needed. Use stepladders rather than a chair to reach high places. Be careful when vacuuming or making the bed, as those tasks can be hard on your lower back.

STRETCHES FOR HOUSECLEANING/LIFTING

Seated Knee to Chest, page 88

Sit & Reach, page 103

Inner Thigh Stretch, page 101

Rear Calf Stretch, page 119

Ankle Circle, page 124

Heel Raise/Heel Drop, page 123

Finger Tap, page 76

Shoulder Roll, page 57

Double Wood Chop, page 53

Picture Frame, page 61

Long Drive or Plane Flight

A long drive or plane flight can cause muscles to get tight. Often the upper and lower back start to ache, and the shoulders and lower legs will get cramped. Sitting for a long time will not only make you inflexible but can be hazardous to your health. There is a condition called "economy class" syndrome, when people sit for a prolonged period; the worst-case scenario is death. Get up as often as possible, drink water, avoid alcohol, and stretch regularly.

STRETCHES FOR LONG DRIVES OR PLANE FLIGHTS

Tennis Watcher, page 44

Turtle, page 46

Head Tilt, page 43

Standing Hip Flexor, page 97

Rear Calf Stretch, page 119

Gas Pedal, page 122

Heel Raise/Heel Drop, page 123

Seated Wrist Stretch, page 70

Finger Tap, page 76

Finger Spreader, page 77

Shoulder Box, page 56

Shoulder Roll, page 57

Shoveling Snow

Anyone who has ever shoveled snow knows how tough this task can be. How often do you pick up the paper to read about someone dying because of shoveling snow? Shoveling is hard on the whole body, but especially your lower back. Always warm up first. Don't hurry or strain—doing so could kill you! This may be an activity that's you should hire a kid to do, rather than doing it yourself and then paying a doctor to fix your back or heart attack. If you feel that your heart and breathing rate are elevated as you're shoveling, stop and check them. If they are high, slow down or stop.

STRETCHES FOR SHOVELING SNOW

Side Bend, page 81

Sit & Reach, page 103

Roll into a Ball, page 91

Standing Hip Flexor, page 97

Heel Raise/Heel Drop, page 123

Apple Picker, page 52

Double Wood Chop, page 53

Windmill, page 50

Mad Cat, page 128

Working at a Desk or Computer

Sitting still and doing anything for a long time is not good for the body. Sitting over a computer causes you to have rounded shoulders, a protruding head, and wrist problems. Get up and move around as often as possible. Stand while on the phone. Walk to deliver a message whenever possible. Set your computer alarm to remind you to get up once every hour. Drink plenty of water or juice to make you get up often. At lunch, don't work at your desk—take a walk. Park as far away from your office as you can, and take the stairs when possible.

If you, like many older adults, find yourself spending hours in one position (at a desk or in an airplane seat, for example), you may feel tired and stiff. The following is a simple way to stay limber:

- get up and walk around

- slowly look left and right

- squeeze your shoulder blades together

- sit in your chair, place your legs straight out in front of you, and reach forward toward your toes.

- reach for the sky several times

STRETCHES FOR WORKING AT A DESK OR COMPUTER

Tennis Watcher, page 44

Side Bend, page 81

Standing Hip Flexor, page 97

Rear Calf Stretch, page 119

Finger Tap, page 76

Apple Picker, page 52

Double Wood Chop, page 53

Mad Cat, page 128

Foot Massage, page 127

Hamstring Massage, page 110

Forearm Massage, page 73

PART THREE

Stretches

Head Tilt

Target: neck

You can also try this stretch sitting with proper posture.

1. Stand with proper posture. While inhaling slowly through your nose, slowly tilt your head toward your left shoulder. Keep your shoulders down and relaxed. Exhale slowly through your lips and hold this position for a moment, feeling the stretch.

2. Now inhale slowly through your nose and slowly tilt your head to your right shoulder. Exhale slowly through your lips and hold this position for a moment, feeling the stretch.

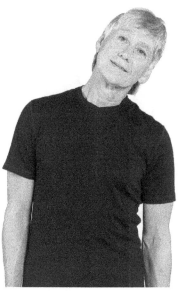

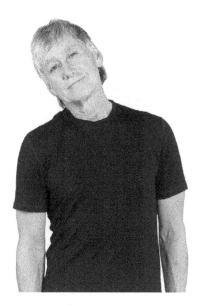

Repeat as desired.

Tennis Watcher

Target: neck

You can also try this stretch sitting with proper posture.

1. Stand with proper posture. While inhaling slowly through your nose, look to your left as far as you can without feeling discomfort. Exhale slowly through your lips and hold this position for a moment, feeling the stretch.

2. Inhale slowly through your nose and look slowly to the right. Exhale slowly through your lips and hold this position for a moment, feeling the stretch.

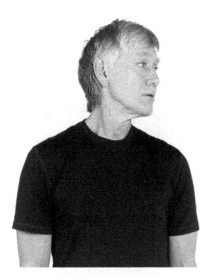

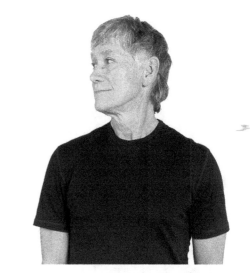

Repeat as desired.

Skyscraper

Target: neck

CAUTION: Avoid hyperextending and hyperflexing the neck. If you have a history of neck problems, do not do this move. You can also try this stretch sitting with proper posture.

1. Stand with proper posture. Position your chin so that it's parallel with the floor. While inhaling slowly through your nose, tilt your head just slightly to look up at the ceiling. Don't arch your neck. Hold this position for a moment, feeling the stretch.

2. Exhale through your lips and lower your chin to your chest just slightly.

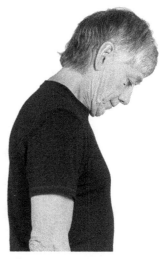

Repeat as many times as feels comfortable.

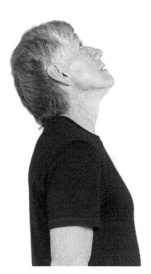

Turtle

Target: neck

This exercise is designed to reverse the effects of "forward" head, a common result of sitting in front of a computer for hours. You can also try this stretch sitting with proper posture.

1. Stand with proper posture. Pretend you're holding an apple under your chin, or keep your chin parallel with the floor. Inhale deeply.

2. While exhaling through your lips, push your chin forward.

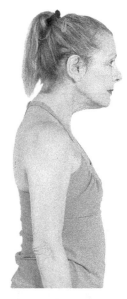

Now inhale through your nose and slowly pull your head back to the neutral position. The focus of this exercise is to pull the head back.

Repeat this move as many times as feels comfortable.

Hold/Relax Turtle

Target: neck

This exercise is designed to reverse the effects of "forward" head, a common result of sitting in front of a computer for hours. You can also try this stretch standing with proper posture.

1. Sit with proper posture. Pretend you're holding an apple under your chin, or position your chin so that it's parallel with the floor. Position the fingertips of your right hand on the center of your forehead. Focus on your deep breathing techniques. Gently press your forehead into your fingertips. Stay mindful of your breathing and hold this position for a comfortable moment.

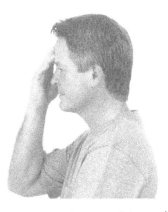

2. Return to starting position, then place your right hand on the back of your head.

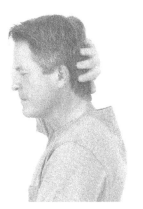

3. Now inhale deeply through your nose and push your skull into your hand. Place more emphasis on this phase of the exercise. Stay mindful of your breathing and hold this position for a comfortable moment.

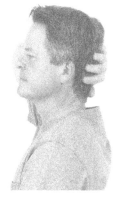

Release and return to starting position.

Variation: Instead of using your fingertips, you can press your head into a pillow held in your hand. If your right shoulder is tight, use your left hand, and vice versa.

Neck Pull/Head Tilt

Target: neck

CAUTION: If you have a history of neck problems (e.g., herniated discs, arthritis of the neck), consult a health professional before performing this move. You can also try this stretch standing with proper posture.

1. Sit with proper posture. While inhaling deeply through your nose, slowly tilt your head to the left.

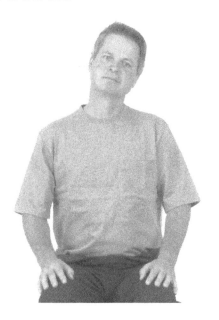

2. Once in this position, place the fingertips of your left hand on the right side of your head. While exhaling through your lips, gently pull your head to your left shoulder. Keep your shoulders relaxed and down. Hold this position and continue to breathe deeply in through your nose and out through your lips.

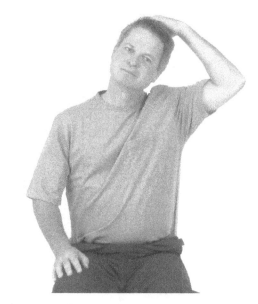

Release and return to starting position.

Repeat on the other side.

Neck Massage

Target: neck

1. Lie on your back with your knees bent, feet on the floor, and arms along your sides. Position a roam roller under the base of your head. Slowly breathe in through your nose and out through your mouth as you allow your back to settle and relax.

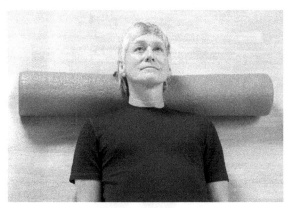

2. Inhale as you gently and slowly look to the left.

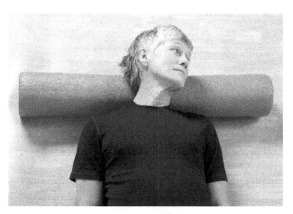

3. Exhale as you return to starting position. Inhale as you look to the right.

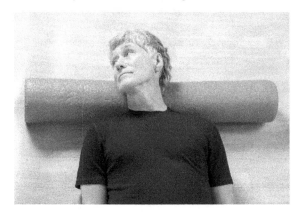

Exhale as you return to starting position.

Windmill

Target: shoulder region

1. Stand with proper posture with your arms at your sides, palms facing forward. Inhale deeply through your nose and slowly raise your arms out to the sides as high as is comfortable. Try to touch your thumbs.

2. Exhale and slowly lower your arms.

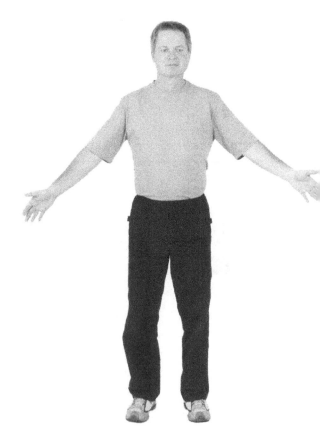

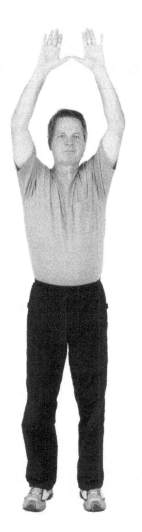

Repeat as desired.

Variation: This exercise can also be done one arm at a time.

Windmill on Roller

Target: shoulder girdle

This exercise increases the range of motion in your shoulder and helps stabilize your muscles. Note that this is a more advanced move and makes use of a foam roller.

1. Lie on a foam roller, resting your head and the entire length of your back on it. Bend your knees and place your feet on the floor; place your arms on the floor alongside your body for balance. Breathe naturally and allow adequate time for your chest and shoulder region to relax and open up. For many people, this is an adequate stretch and it's OK to stop here without progressing to the following steps.

2. Once comfortable and stable, extend both arms up to the ceiling while maintaining balance on the roller; your palms should face each other. Be sure to stabilize your core the entire time by contracting your abs.

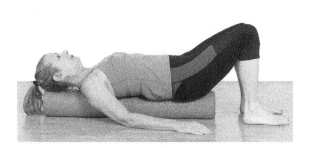

3. Allow one arm to move forward and the other backward. Stay within your comfortable range of motion.

Reverse directions.

Release and relax.

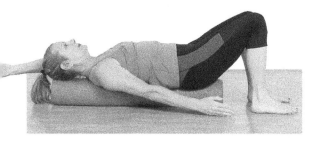

Apple Picker

Target: deltoids

1. Stand with proper posture and place your hands on your shoulders. Reach your right hand as high upward as is comfortable.

2. Place the right hand back on your shoulder. Now reach up with your left hand.

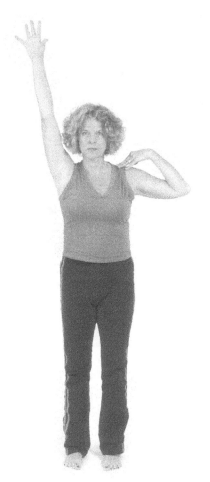

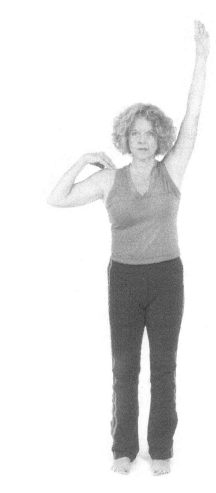

Repeat as desired.

Double Wood Chop

Target: deltoids

1. Stand with proper posture. Position your hands in front of your body and interlace your fingers.

2. Inhale deeply through your nose and slowly raise both arms in front of you to a comfortable height. Hold 1 to 2 seconds.

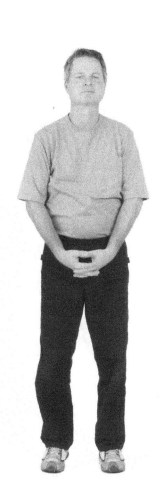

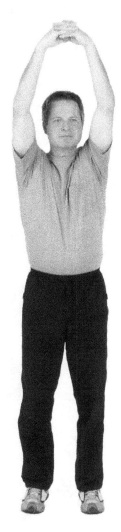

Slowly lower your arms to starting position.

Repeat as desired.

Soup Can Pour

Target: deltoids, rotator cuff

1. Stand with proper posture, your arms at your side and your palms facing back. Inhale deeply through your nose and bring both arms slightly forward as your raise them out to the sides, keeping your palm facing back. Raise your arms no higher than shoulder level.

2. Exhale as you lower your arms.

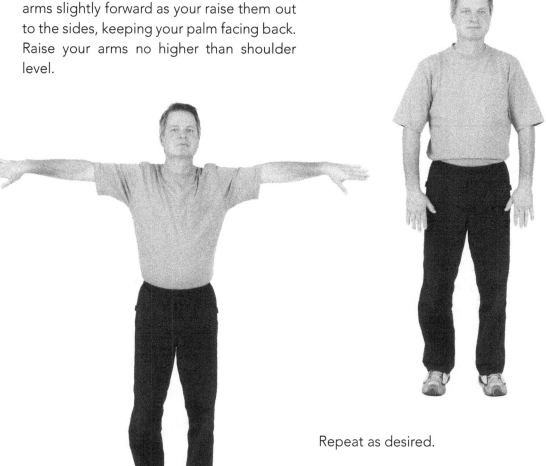

Repeat as desired.

Rotator Cuff

Target: deltoids, rotator cuff

You can substitute a rolled-up towel for the block.

1. Stand with proper posture with your arms at your sides and squeeze a block between your right arm and your torso. Bend your right elbow 90 degrees and point your thumb up.

2. Keeping your elbow as close to your body as possible and your forearm parallel to the floor, rotate your forearm out to the side.

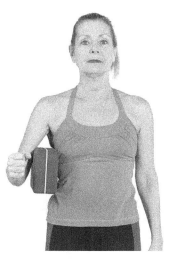

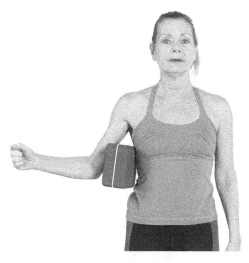

Rotate your forearm back in toward your body. Repeat as desired then switch sides.

Variation: Try this with your palm facing down or up.

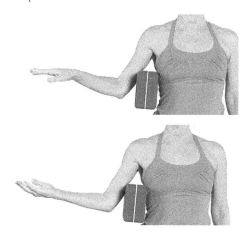

Shoulder Box

Target: shoulders, trapezius

1. Stand with proper posture. Inhaling deeply through your nose, slowly lift up your shoulders.

2. Now pull your shoulders back and squeeze the shoulder blades together and down.

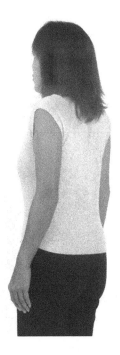

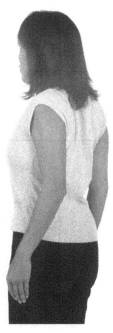

Exhaling through your lips, drop your shoulders and return to starting position.

Repeat as desired.

Shoulder Roll

Target: shoulders, trapezius

You can also try this stretch standing with proper posture.

1. Sit with proper posture in a stable chair. Inhale slowly and deeply through your nose. Exhaling through your nose, roll your shoulders forward, attempting to touch your shoulders together.

2. Now inhale and focus on squeezing your shoulder blades together, moving your shoulders back and opening up your chest.

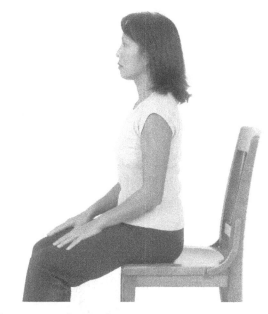

Repeat as desired.

Prone Reverse Fly

Target: shoulders, trapezius

1. Carefully lie facedown on a half foam roller with its flat side down; your toes should rest on the ground. Extend your arms out to your sides in a "T."

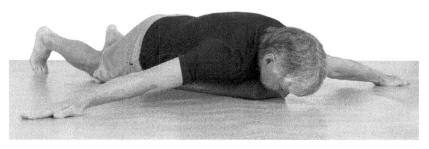

2. Keeping your abs tight, slowly lift your arms a comfortable distance off the floor. Hold.

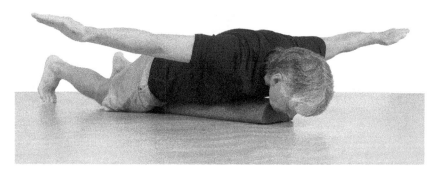

Return to starting position.

Over the Top

Target: shoulders, rotator cuff

You can also try this stretch standing with proper posture.

1. Sit with proper posture in a stable chair. Raise your right arm and place your hand on your back, over your right shoulder.

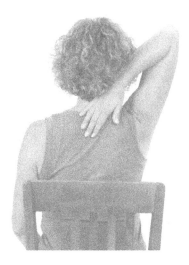

2. Place your left hand on your right elbow and gently press your right arm down your back as far as feels comfortable. Hold the position for a comfortable moment.

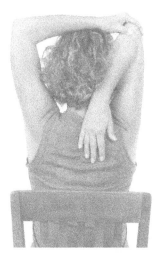

Switch sides and repeat.

Variation: In Step 2, press your right arm down as you push your right elbow up into your hand. Hold this position for a comfortable moment, remembering to breathe. Then release and allow your hand to slide a little farther down your back.

Choker

Target: shoulders, rotator cuff

You can also try this stretch standing with proper posture.

1. Sit with proper posture in a stable chair. Place your right hand on your left shoulder.

2. Place your left hand on your right elbow and gently press your right elbow toward your throat. Hold for a comfortable moment.

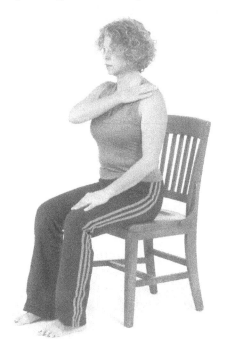

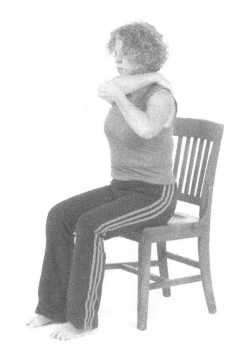

Switch sides and repeat.

Variation: In Step 2, press your right elbow into your left hand. Hold for a comfortable moment, remembering to breathe. Then release to reach the right hand a little farther back.

Picture Frame

Target: shoulders

Remember not to let your lower back arch. You can also try this stretch sitting with proper posture.

1. Stand with proper posture. Place your right hand on your left elbow and your left hand on your right elbow.

2. Slowly lift your arms overhead, raising your arms as high as feels comfortable. Hold the position for a moment. You are now framing your face in a picture frame created by your arms—smile!

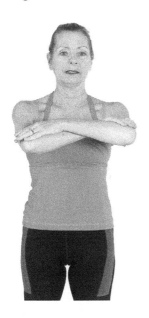

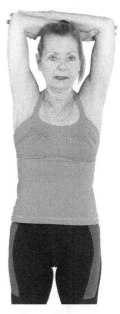

Repeat as desired.

The Zipper

Target: shoulders

You can also try this stretch sitting with proper posture.

1. Stand with proper posture. Hold a strap in your right hand and raise your arm above your head. Bring your right hand down behind your head and grab the dangling end of the strap with your left hand.

2. Raise your right hand up as high as possible to lift the lower hand, staying in your pain-free zone. Hold the position for a comfortable moment.

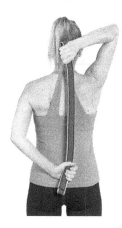

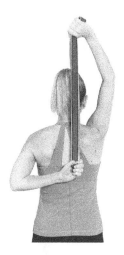

3. Pull down with your left hand to bring down the right hand. Hold the position for a comfortable moment.

Advanced: As you become more flexible, eliminate the use of the strap and try to grab your fingertips.

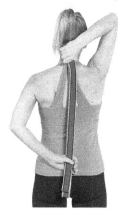

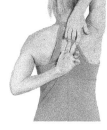

Switch sides and repeat.

I, Y, & T

Target: shoulders

1. Sit on a stability ball and then slowly move your feet forward until the ball is comfortably supporting your upper back, neck, and head. Your feet should be shoulder-width apart and bent 90 degrees. Extend your arms toward the ceiling with palms facing each other.

2. While engaging your core muscles, slowly and deliberately take both arms back by your ears, making your body look like an "I" from a bird's-eye view.

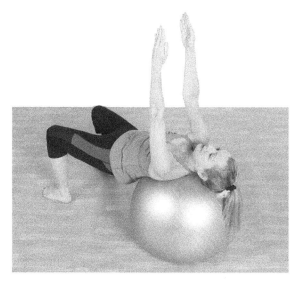

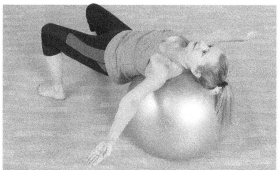

3. Return to starting position and then slightly take your arms back and to the sides, as if making a "Y."

4. Return to starting position and then open your arms out to the sides to make a "T."

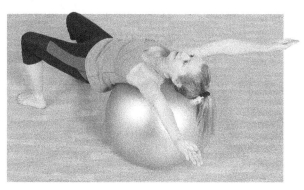

Elbow Touch

Target: chest, shoulder retractor

You can also try this stretch standing with proper posture.

1. Sit with proper posture in a stable chair. Place your hands on your shoulders, elbows pointing forward.

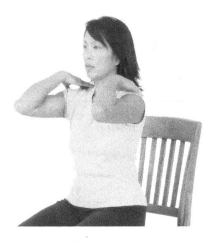

2. Slowly bring your elbows together in front of your body.

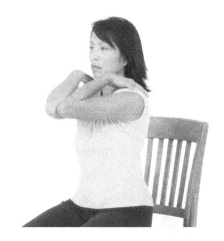

3. Bring your elbows back and squeeze your shoulder blades together. Hold for a moment, focusing on opening up your chest.

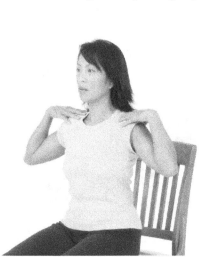

Bring your elbows back to the starting position and repeat as desired.

Variation: Once you've done Step 2, draw circles with your elbows.

Elbow Touch against Wall

Target: chest

1. Stand with your back and head against the wall. Place your hands on your shoulders and point your elbows forward.

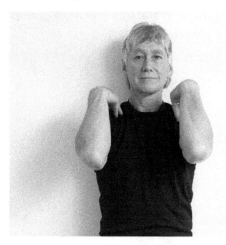

2. Carefully move your elbows toward the wall. Don't arch your back to increase your range. Touching the wall is not critical; the goal is to feel a gentle stretch in your chest and shoulders.

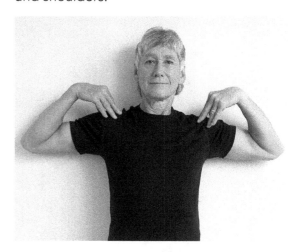

3. Slowly move your elbows back to center until you can touch them together.

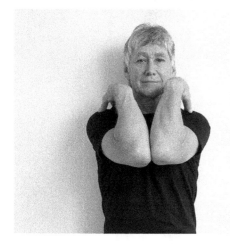

Return to starting position.

Hands behind Back

Target: shoulders, chest

You can also use a bar instead of a strap.

1. Stand with proper posture. Hold the ends of a strap in each hand behind your bottom.

2. Attempt to straighten your arms behind you. Focus on squeezing your shoulder blades together. Hold this position for as long as is comfortable.

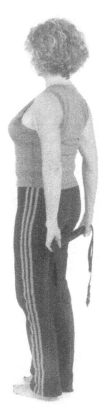

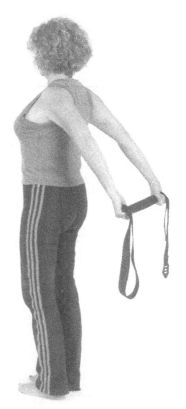

Advanced: Instead of using a strap, interlock your hands behind your back.

Pec Stretch

Target: shoulders, chest

You can also try this stretch standing with proper posture.

1. Sit with proper posture in a stable chair. Place your hands behind your head.

2. Gently move your elbows back and try to bring your shoulder blades together. Focus on opening up the chest and tightening the upper back muscles. Only go as far back as is comfortable and hold for a moment.

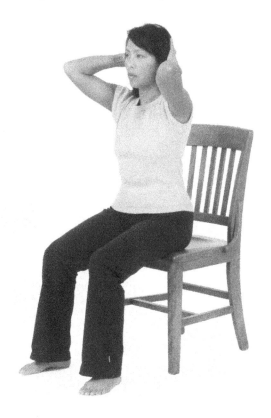

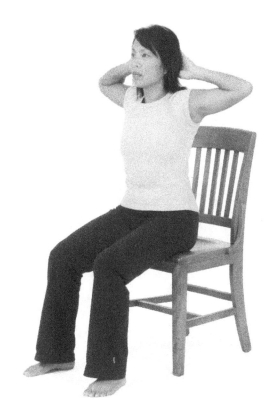

Repeat as desired.

Chest Stretch

Target: chest

CAUTION: Be careful not to extend back too far; stay in your comfort zone.

1. Kneel in front of a stability ball and place your belly and chest on the ball. Rest your hands and forearms on the ball. Extend your legs behind you, making a straight line from head to heels.

2. Keeping your head and neck neutral, gently raise your chest off the ball. Don't come up too high.

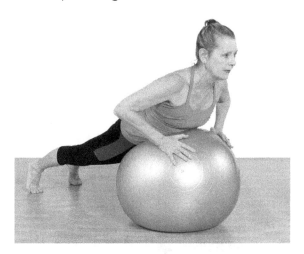

Return to starting position.

Inward/Outward Wrist Stretch

Target: forearms, wrists

1. Sit with proper posture in a stable chair. Rest your fists on your thighs with your thumbs pointing up toward the ceiling.

2. Slowly turn your fists so that your thumbs point inward.

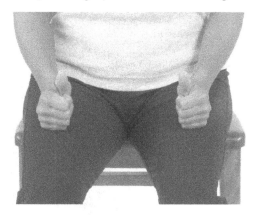

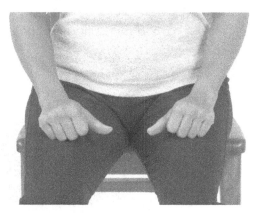

3. Slowly turn your fists so that your thumbs point outward.

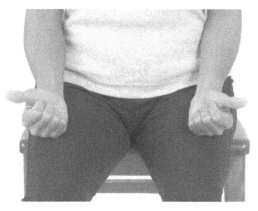

Repeat as desired.

Seated Wrist Stretch

Target: forearm, wrists

1. Sit in a stable chair. Rest your forearms on your thighs so that your wrists hang off. Your hands should be in loose fists. Slowly lift your knuckles toward the ceiling and hold 1 to 2 seconds.

2. Slowly lower your knuckles toward the floor and hold 1 to 2 seconds.

Repeat as feels comfortable.

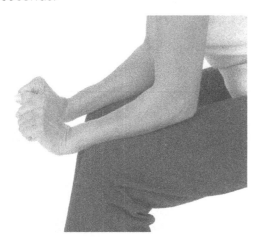

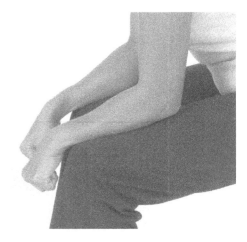

Advanced Variation: After you lift your knuckles upward in Step 1, extend your fingertips, then make a fist, lower your knuckles, and extend your fingers downward.

Standing Wrist Stretch

Target: forearm, wrists

The Position: Stand with proper posture. Extend your right arm in front of you to shoulder height, with your palm facing forward and fingers pointing toward the ceiling. Gently pull your fingers back with your left hand until a desired stretch is felt under your wrist. Hold the stretch for several seconds.

Advanced Variation: Try doing the exercise with the fingertips pointing down.

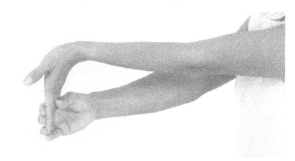

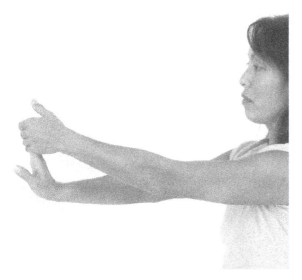

Repeat as desired then switch sides.

Kneeling Wrist Stretch

Target: forearms, wrists

This is a very advanced exercise.

1. Kneel on the floor, using a mat as necessary.

2. Slowly place your fingers on the floor so that your fingers are pointing toward you.

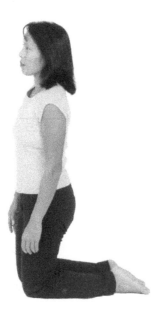

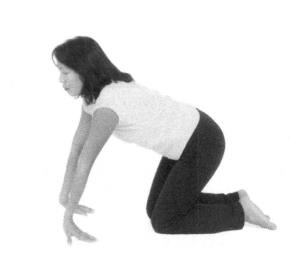

3. Slowly lower your palms to the floor without discomfort in your wrists. Be sure to keep your elbows soft. Hold the stretch for a comfortable moment.

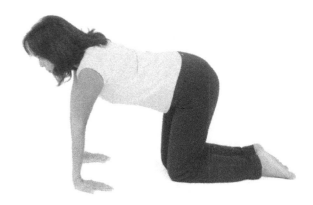

Forearm Massage

Target: forearms

The Position: Kneel in front of a foam roller and place your forearms on the roller with your palms down. Slowly move your arms forward and back across the roller. Along the way, stop and apply pressure wherever additional attention is needed.

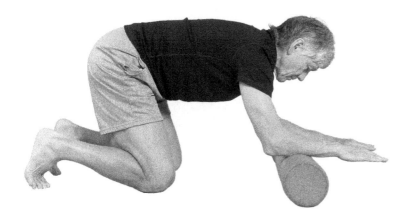

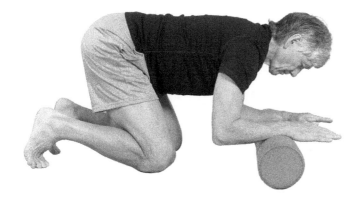

Band Roll-Up

Target: forearm, fingers

1. Sit with proper posture on a stability ball. Hold the end of a resistance band in your right hand and extend the right arm straight out in front of you, palm down.

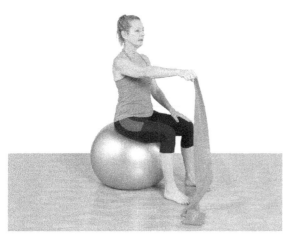

2. Turn your palm up and grab more band in your hand.

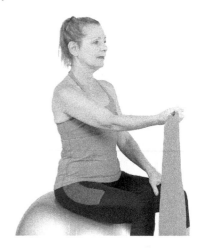

3. Turn your palm down and grab more band, balling up the band in your hand as you go. Continue until you've grabbed as much band as you can, then squeeze tightly several times.

Switch hands and repeat.

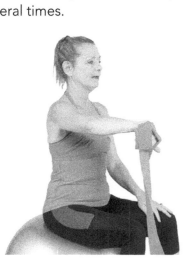

Squeezer

Target: forearm, fingers

1. Sit with proper posture in a chair. Hold a small, soft, squeezable object in your right hand and extend that arm straight out in front of you. Keep your left arm by your side.

2. Slowly squeeze the object and hold for 1 to 2 seconds.

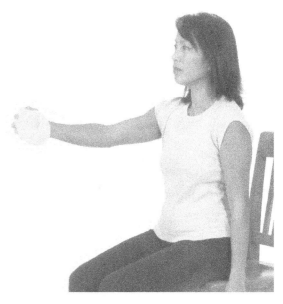

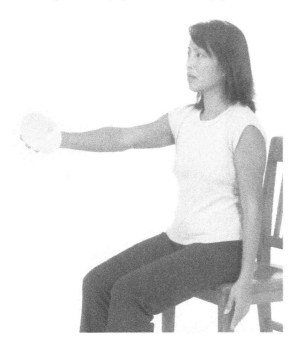

Repeat until the hand has done a comfortable number.

Switch hands and repeat.

Modification: You can also try doing this with an object in both hands.

Variation: Try this on something more difficult to squeeze, like a tennis ball.

Finger Tap

Target: hands, forearms, fingers

1. Sit at the edge of a stable chair. Rest your hands on your thighs with your palms turned up. Touch the tip of your little finger to your thumb then progress through each finger until you reach your index finger.

2. Now turn your palms down and repeat the exercise.

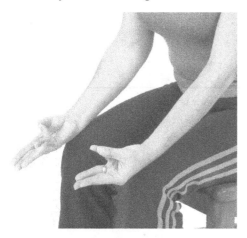

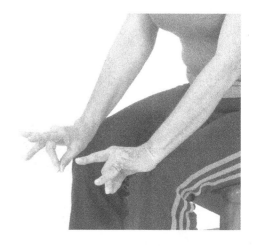

Finger Base Tap Variation: Touch the thumb to the base of your little finger, then progress through each finger until you reach the index finger. Now turn your palms down and repeat the exercise.

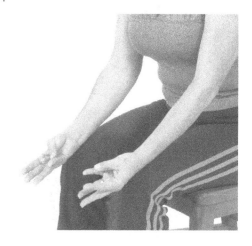

Finger Spreader

Target: hands, forearms, fingers

This exercise can also be done standing.

1. Sit with proper posture in a stable chair. Rest your hands on your thighs with your palms down and fingers gently spread. Pinch your fingers and thumb together.

2. Now separate all fingers and thumb as far apart as possible.

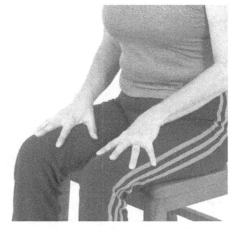

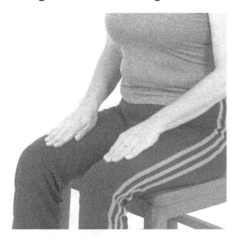

Turn your palms up and repeat steps 1 and 2.

V-W Stretch

Target: hands, fingers

This exercise can also be done standing.

1. Sit with proper posture in a stable chair. Rest your hands on your thighs with your palms down. Squeeze all your fingers together.

2. Separate one finger at a time, starting with the little finger, then the ring finger, until you've separated all your fingers. Squeeze your fingers together and repeat the exercise.

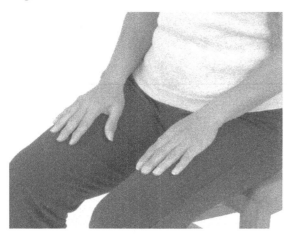

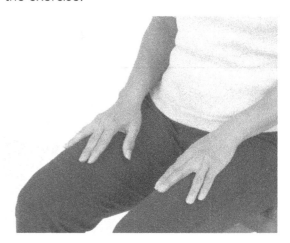

Advanced Variation: Increase the challenge by holding your arms straight out in front of you. Instead of just separating your fingers, try to make a V and W. To make a V: Spread your little finger and ring finger away from your index finger and middle finger. To make a W: Put your ring finger and middle finger together and separate the little finger and index finger from the group.

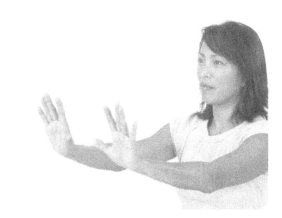

Palm Tree

Target: torso

CAUTION: If you have poor balance or lower back problems, avoid this move. You can also try this stretch standing with proper posture.

1. Sit with proper posture in a stable chair. Raise your hands overhead with your arms as straight as feels comfortable. Inhale deeply through your nose. While exhaling through your lips, slowly lean to your left. Hold the position for a comfortable moment, feeling the stretch along the right side of your body.

2. Now inhale fully and deeply through your nose and lean to your right. Hold this position for a comfortable moment.

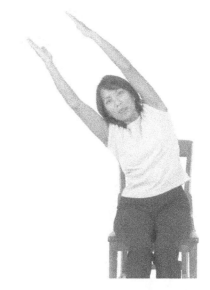

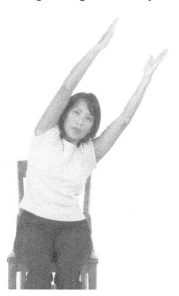

Advanced: Try pressing your hands together as you do the side bends.

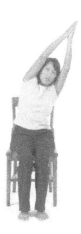

Twister

Target: torso

CAUTION: Be careful if you have lower back problems.

You can also try this stretch standing with proper posture.

1. Sit with proper posture in a stable chair. Cross your arms in front of your chest and inhale slowly and deeply through your nose. While exhaling through your lips, slowly twist to your left. Hold the position for a comfortable moment and feel the stretch in your torso.

2. Inhale and return to the starting position before exhaling and twisting to your right. Hold the position for a comfortable moment and feel the stretch in your torso.

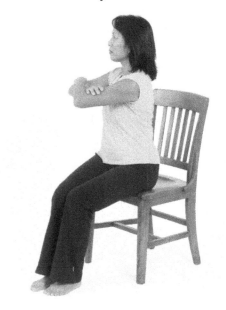

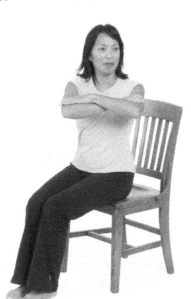

Variation: Rest a broom handle across the back of your shoulders and perform smoothly and gently.

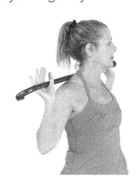

Side Bend

Target: torso

CAUTION: Be careful if you have lower back pain. You can also try this stretch sitting with proper posture.

1. Stand with proper posture. Raise your right arm over your head to a comfortable height. Inhale deeply through your nose.

2. Now exhale through your lips and slowly and carefully lean to the left. Once you have leaned over enough to feel a gentle stretch along the right side of your body, hold this position for a comfortable moment.

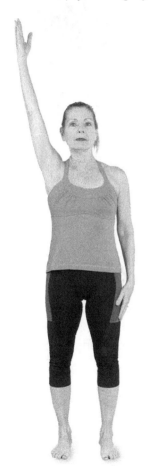

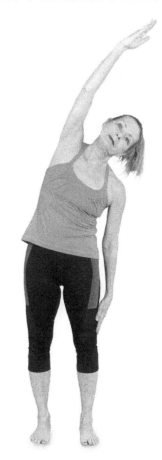

Switch sides and repeat.

Variation: If your shoulder is stiff, place your hand on top of your head.

Side Bend with Band

Target: torso

CAUTION: Be careful if you have arthritis of the spine.

1. Stand with your feet shoulder-width apart and place a band under your right foot. Grasp the band near your right hip with your right hand.

2. Lean your body to the left.

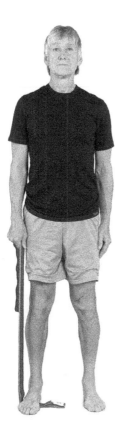

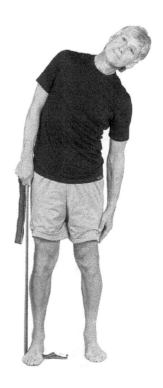

Return to start position and repeat.

Switch sides.

Torso Rotation

Target: torso

This exercise makes use of a resistance band to increase the stretch and strengthen the torso.

1. Secure the band to a door with the proper strap so that the band is at chest height. While standing with your left side to the door, grab the band with both hands and move away from the door until your arms are fully extended. Stand with your feet shoulder-width apart.

2. Slowly twist to the right and hold for 1 to 2 seconds.

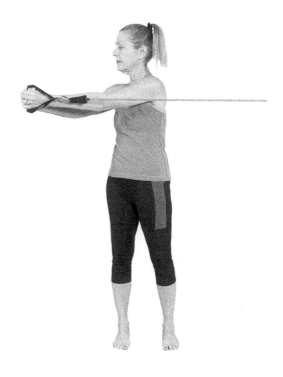

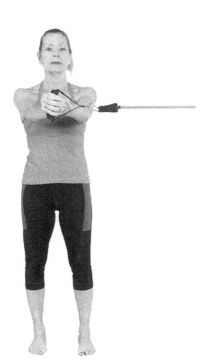

Return to start position and repeat as desired.

Switch sides.

Torso Relax

Target: torso, spine, neck

This releases back tension and lengthens the spine and neck. Use a large stability ball.

CAUTION: If you're pregnant or have stomach issues, speak to your health professional before doing this movement.

The Position: Kneel in front of a stability ball. Drape your upper body over the ball, hugging the ball or placing your hands on the floor in front of you as necessary. Breathe slowly and fully.

To get off the ball, shift your weight back toward your hips so that you return to kneeling.

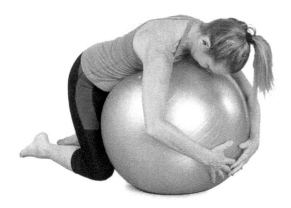

Knee Roll

Target: torso, hips

CAUTION: If you have lower back problems, avoid this move.

1. Lie on a mat with your knees bent and your feet flat on the floor. Place your arms straight out to your sides in a "T" position. While inhaling through your nose, allow your knees to drop gently to the right without discomfort. Exhale and hold this position for a comfortable moment.

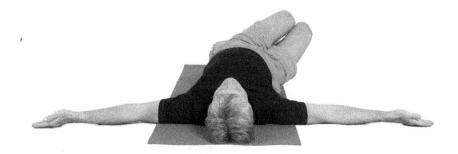

2. Inhale and bring your knees back to center, then gently drop them to your left. Exhale and hold this position for a comfortable moment.

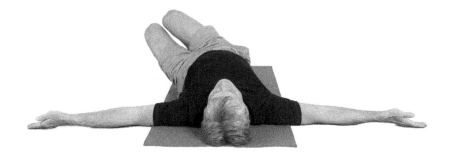

Cross-Leg Drop

Target: torso, piriformis

CAUTION: Be careful if you have lower back problems.

1. Lie on a mat with your knees bent and your feet flat on the floor. While focusing on your breathing, place your left knee on top of your right knee.

2. Slowly allow your left knee to gently fall toward the right side. Stop when you feel tightness. Hold this position for a comfortable moment. The stretch should be felt near the rear pocket area of the left leg. Focus on the stretch, not on how close you can bring your knees to the floor.

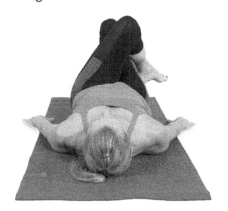

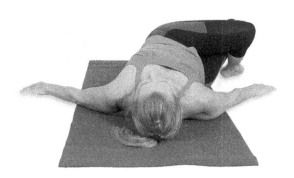

Switch sides and repeat.

Diagonal Knee to Chest

Target: torso, gluteus maximus

CAUTION: Avoid this stretch if you have hip problems.

1. Lie on a mat with your knees bent and your feet flat on the floor. Place your right knee on top of your left knee.

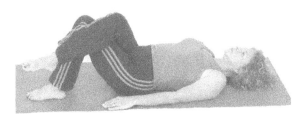

2. Draw your knees in toward your chest and pull your right knee toward your left shoulder using your left hand. Hold for a comfortable moment, focusing on the sensation of the stretch, not on how close your knee comes to your shoulder.

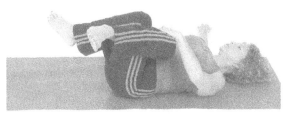

Switch sides and repeat.

Variation: You can also use a strap to draw in your knees.

Seated Knee to Chest

Target: lower back, gluteus maximus

1. Sit with proper posture in a stable chair and place your feet on the floor. Clasp both hands beneath your left leg.

2. Bring your left knee toward your chest. Hold this position for a comfortable moment, feeling the stretch in the gluteal region.

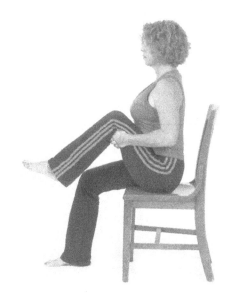

Release the knee, switch sides, and repeat.

Single Knee to Chest

Target: lower back, gluteus maximus

1. Lie on a mat and, if needed, place a pillow under your head. Bend your knees and place both feet flat on the floor. Loop a strap behind the back of your right leg and hold an end of the strap in each hand.

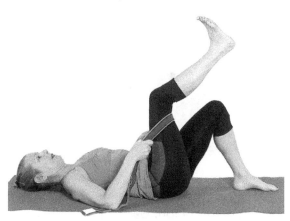

2. Gently pull the straps to bring the knee toward your chest. Hold this stretch for a comfortable moment.

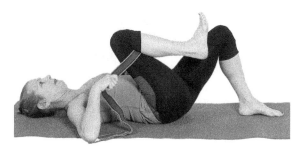

Release the knee, switch sides, and repeat.

Intermediate Variation: This can also be done using just the hands to bring in the knee.

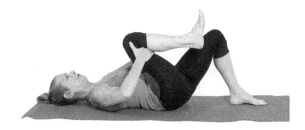

Advanced Variation: Extend one leg straight on the floor and bring one knee to your chest.

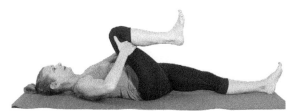

Double Knee to Chest

Target: lower back, gluteus maximus

1. Lie on a mat and, if needed, place a pillow under your head. Bend your knees and place both feet flat on the floor. Loop a strap behind the backs of both legs and hold an end of the strap in each hand.

2. Gently pull the straps to bring your knees to your chest. Hold this position for a comfortable moment, feeling the stretch in your bottom and lower back.

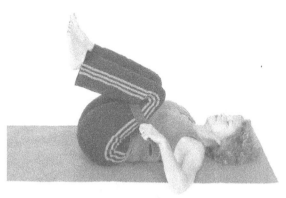

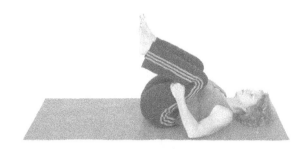

Advanced Variation: Use just your hands to draw in your knees.

Roll into a Ball

Target: lower back, gluteus maximus, torso

CAUTION: Do not do this stretch if you have knee problems.

1. Place your hands and knees on the floor. Inhale through your nose.

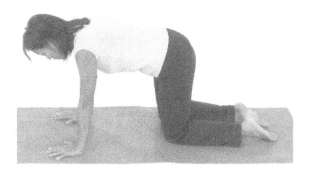

2. While exhaling deeply through your mouth, slowly allow your bottom to drop toward your heels. If you feel discomfort, you may place a pillow between your heels and bottom.

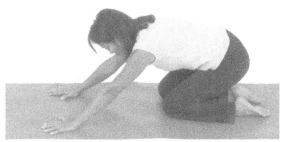

3. Place your forehead on the floor or a pillow, and position your arms alongside your body. Hold this position for a comfortable moment, enjoying the sensation of the stretch up and down your back.

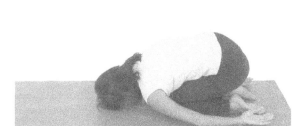

Variation: If you can find a friend to rub up and down your back while doing this stretch, it will enhance the stretch.

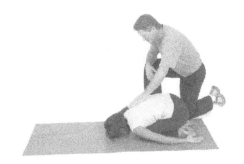

Advanced Variation: Stretch your arms out straight in front of you.

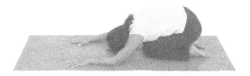

Piriformis Stretch

Target: lower back, piriformis

The piriformis muscle is a deep-lying muscle in the gluteal region, through which the sciatic nerve passes. When the piriformis is too tight, it can cramp the sciatic nerve, causing the symptoms of sciatica.

1. Lie on a mat with your knees bent and your feet flat on the floor. Cross your right knee on top of your left knee.

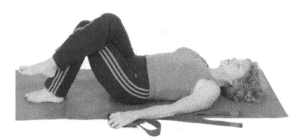

2. Loop a strap around both legs and pull your knees in toward your chest. Stop when tension occurs. Hold this position for a comfortable moment, focusing on the sensation of the stretch.

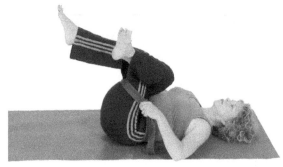

Switch sides and repeat.

Advanced Variation: Use only your hands to pull your knees in.

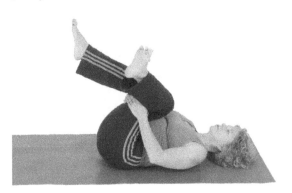

Rock 'n' Roll

Target: lower back, torso

1. Lie on a mat and slowly bring both knees toward your chest. Gently reach around both legs and allow your shoulders to lift off the mat.

2–3. While inhaling deeply through your nose and exhaling through your lips, slowly rock left and right, enjoying the relaxing feeling.

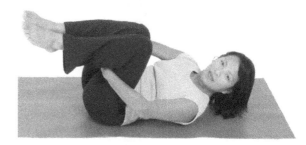

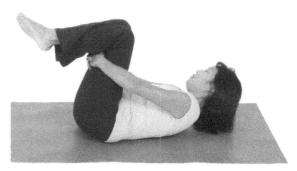

Rock 'n' Roll on Roller

Target: lower back, torso

1. Lie on your back and place a foam roller under your tailbone. Slowly bring both knees toward your chest with your hands.

2–3. While inhaling deeply through your nose and exhaling through your lips, slowly rock left and right, enjoying the relaxing feeling.

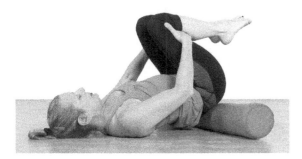

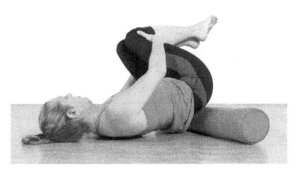

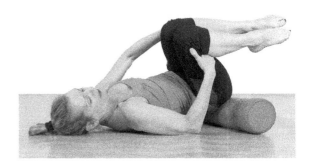

Ab Stretch

Target: abdominals, lower back, torso

This stretch requires a large stability ball and a medium-sized therapy ball. If you don't have a medium ball, you can use two small therapy balls, firm or hard. Placing both your fists (instead of balls) under your back also works.

The Position: Lie on your back and place your legs on top of a stability ball. If you can tolerate it, place a medium-sized therapy ball under your lower back. Place your hands anywhere they're comfortable (along your sides, under your head). Breathe and relax, allowing your abdominal area to elongate.

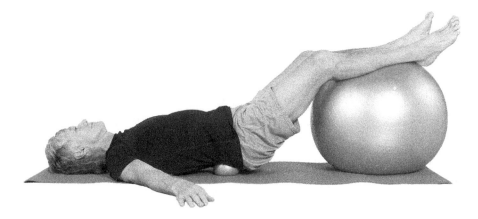

Kneeling Hip Flexor

Target: hip flexors

CAUTION: Avoid this stretch if you have poor balance or bad knees.

The Position: Kneel on a mat with a chair on your right side. Move your right knee forward so that you can place your right foot flat on the floor. Maintain an erect position by pulling in your chin, squeezing your shoulder blades together, pulling in your belly button, and contracting your gluteals.

Slowly press your hips forward until you feel a comfortable stretch in front of your kneeling leg. Hold this stretch for a comfortable moment.

Intermediate Variation: Slide your left knee back and press up onto the ball of your foot.

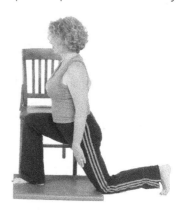

Advanced Variation: You can rise onto the ball of your rear foot to lift your knee off the floor and intensify the stretch.

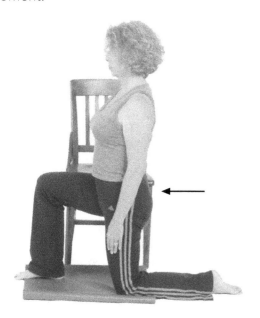

Switch sides and repeat.

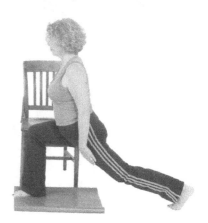

Standing Hip Flexor

Target: hip flexors

The Position: Stand behind a chair and place your hands on the back of the chair. Slide your right leg back a comfortable distance. Keeping your rear heel down, gently tuck your tailbone under and press your hips forward. Hold this stretch for a comfortable moment, focusing on feeling the stretch in the upper leg/hip region rather than in the calf area.

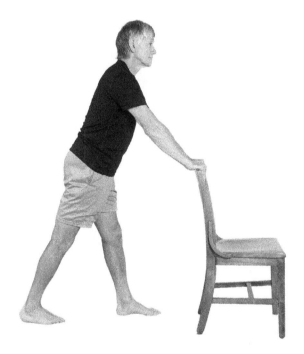

Switch sides and repeat.

Supine Hip Flexor

Target: hip flexors

1. Lie on your back with your knees bent and feet flat on the floor. Place a medium-sized therapy ball under your tailbone. Adjust the ball so that you balance comfortably on it.

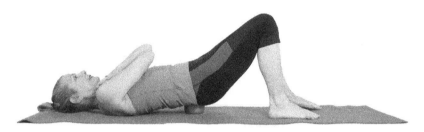

2. Once you've settled your weight into the ball, inhale and bring your right knee to your chest and clasp your hands beneath your knee. Exhale and straighten your left leg as far as is comfortable along the floor. Hold, breathing slowly and fully, feeling the stretch in your extended leg.

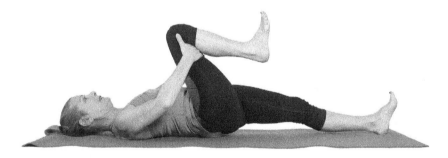

Slowly switch sides.

The Butterfly

Target: inner thighs, lower back

1. Sit on a mat with your knees bent and your feet flat on the floor. Place the soles of your feet together and gently allow your knees to drop to the floor.

2. Loop a strap around your feet and gently pull yourself forward, not down. Hold this stretch for a comfortable moment.

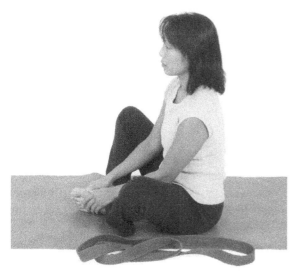

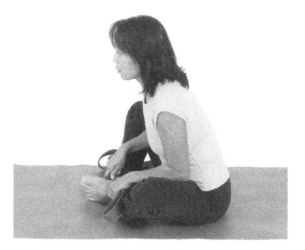

Repeat as desired.

Advanced Variation: Place your hands on your ankles and pull yourself forward.

Seated Inner Thigh Stretch

Target: inner thighs

1. Sit at the edge of a stable chair and place both feet flat on the floor. Spread your legs apart and point your knees and toes 45 degrees out to the sides.

2. Place your hands on the insides of your thighs and gently push your legs a little wider. Hold this stretch for a comfortable moment.

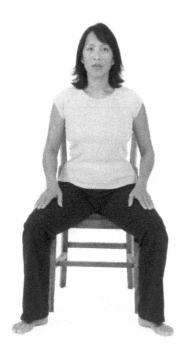 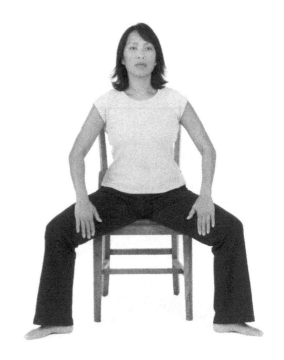

Repeat as desired.

Inner Thigh Stretch

Target: inner thighs

1. Lie on your back with your knees bent and feet flat on the floor. Place a medium-sized therapy ball under your tailbone. Adjust the ball so that you balance comfortably on it.

2. Once you've settled your weight into the ball, exhale, and slowly let your knees drop open to the sides. Hold, breathing slowly and fully, feeling the stretch in your inner thighs.

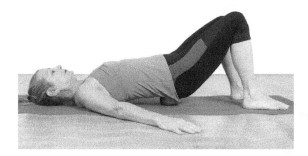

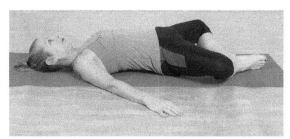

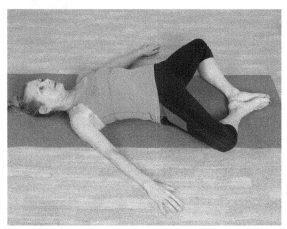

Inner Thigh Massage

Target: inner thighs

1. Resting on your forearms, lie facedown with both legs extended. Bend your right leg and take your knee to the right side, opening up your hip. Place 1 or 2 firm small balls (in a sock) under the inside of your right thigh.

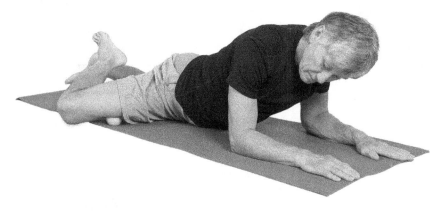

2. Gently roll the ball around under your thigh, controlling the pressure by shifting your weight. Breathe slowly and fully.

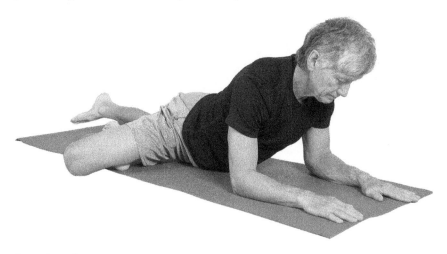

Switch sides.

Sit & Reach

Target: hamstrings

Be careful not to tip the chair over.

1. Sit at the edge of a stable chair. Loop a strap around the ball of your left foot and hold an end of the strap in each hand. Extend your legs straight out in front of you and place your heels on the floor with your toes pointing up 90 degrees.

2. Stack your left heel on top of your right foot, keeping your legs as straight as possible. Inhale deeply through your nose.

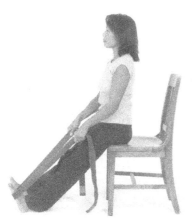

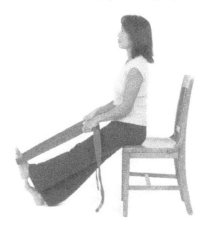

3. Now exhale through your lips and gently pull yourself forward by leading with your chest rather than rounding your back.

Intermediate Variation: Instead of using the strap, you can extend your arms forward and gently reach forward with your fingertips.

Advanced Variation: Place both heels on a chair in front of you.

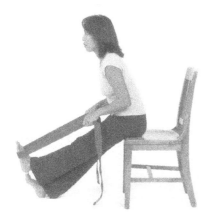

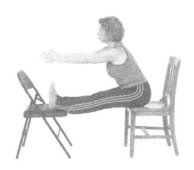

Switch sides and repeat.

Bent-Over Toe Touch

Target: hamstrings

CAUTION: Stop if you notice undue compression in your knee or experience any lower back discomfort. If you feel a cramp coming on, do a hamstring stretch.

1. Stand upright in proper posture with a slight bend in the knees. Slowly bend over from the waist with knees slightly bent and attempt to touch your toes.

2. Stop when you feel tension in the hamstring muscles; place both hands on your thighs to take the load off your lower back. Hold 30 seconds to 1 minute.

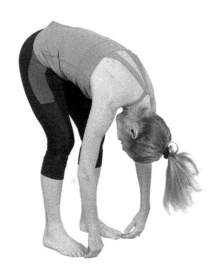

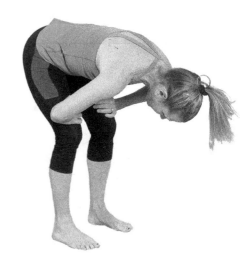

Return to upright posture by slowly rounding your back.

Modification: If you have balance issues, place hands on a chair for support.

Advanced Variation: Cross your right leg over your left leg and perform the stretch, then try with your left leg over your right.

V Stretch

Target: hamstrings, inner thighs

1. Sit on a mat with both legs extended into a "V" position. Inhale deeply.

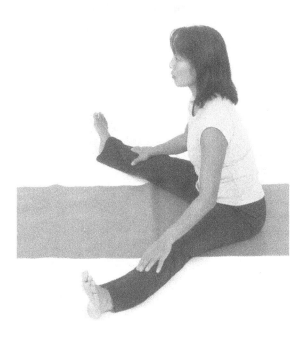

2. While keeping your head and torso tall, exhale and allow yourself to fall forward until you feel a comfortable stretch in the hamstrings and inner thighs. Be sure not to round your back. Hold this stretch for a comfortable moment, focusing on the sensation of the stretch, not on going as far as possible. Inhale through your nose and return to the starting position.

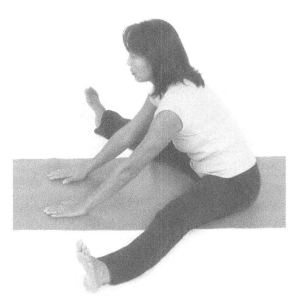

Straight-Leg Stretch

Target: hamstrings, lower back

1. Sit at the edge of a stable chair and place both feet flat on the floor. Position a strap around the sole of the left foot and hold an end of the strap in each hand.

2. Inhale deeply through your nose and straighten your left leg. Now exhale through your lips and attempt to straighten your left leg as far as is comfortable. Hold this position for a comfortable moment.

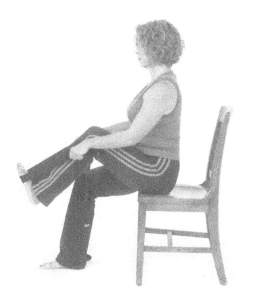

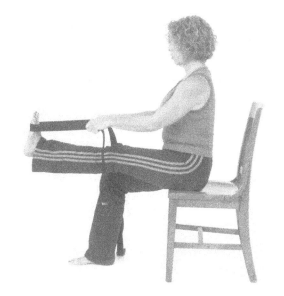

Switch sides and repeat.

Advanced Variation: Place one heel on a chair in front of you.

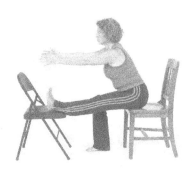

Inverted Figure 4

Target: hamstrings

1. Lie on a mat with your knees bent and your feet flat on the floor. Place your left ankle on top of your right knee. Inhale deeply through your nose.

2. Wrap both hands around your right leg and bring your knee and ankle to your chest while exhaling.

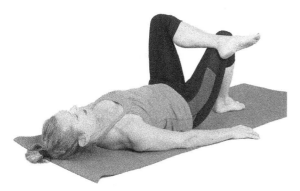

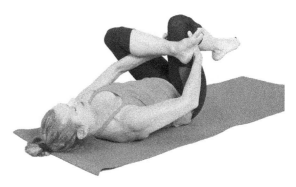

3. Now straighten your right leg toward the ceiling as much as is comfortable. Focus on inhaling and exhaling fully and hold this stretch for a comfortable moment.

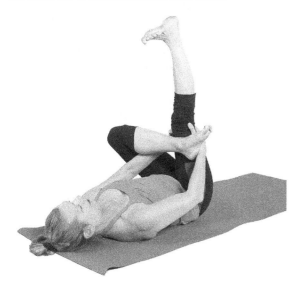

Switch sides and repeat.

Figure 4

Target: hamstrings, lower back

CAUTION: Avoid this move if you have knee problems.

1. Sit on a mat with both legs extended straight out in front of you. Keep your torso as tall as possible. Place your left foot against your right knee. Loop a strap around the sole of your right foot and hold on to the ends of the strap. Inhale deeply through your nose.

2. While keeping your head and torso tall, exhale and pull yourself forward until you feel a comfortable stretch in the backs of your legs. Hold this stretch for a comfortable moment, focusing on the sensation of the stretch, not on going as far as possible. The goal is to hold the stretch for 60 seconds. Exhale through your lips and return to the starting position.

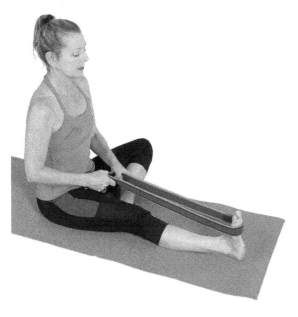

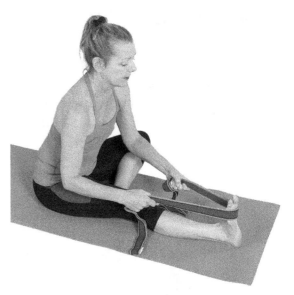

Switch sides and repeat.

Hamstring/Hip Release

Target: hamstrings, lower back, hips

1. Lie on your back with your knees bent and feet flat on the floor. Place a medium-sized therapy ball under your tailbone. Adjust the ball so that you balance comfortably on it. Inhale and bring your knees to your chest and then exhale and extend your legs up to the ceiling, as if sliding your legs up an imaginary wall.

2. Keeping your legs together, gently shift your weight to your right hip. Hold, feeling the stretch in your hip.

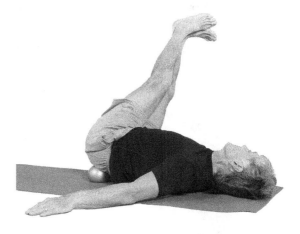

3. Gently shift your weight to your left hip and hold. Repeat as necessary.

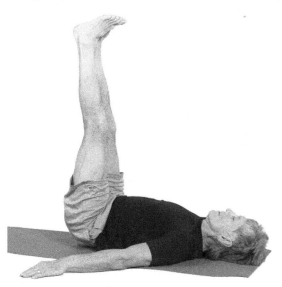

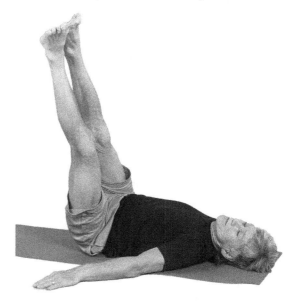

Hamstring Massage

Target: hamstrings

The Position: Sit upright in a chair and place 1 or 2 firm balls (in a sock) under the back of one leg. Roll the ball around under your thigh, from above your knee to under your buttock, controlling the pressure by shifting your weight. Use your intuition to guide you on how hard to press and where and how long to roll. Breathe slowly and fully.

Variation: If rolling the ball is too painful, try slowly extending the leg, staying mindful of the pressure.

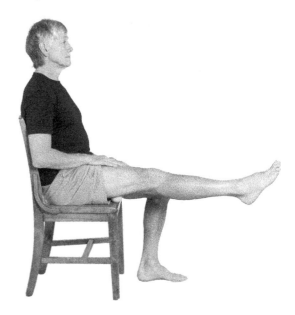

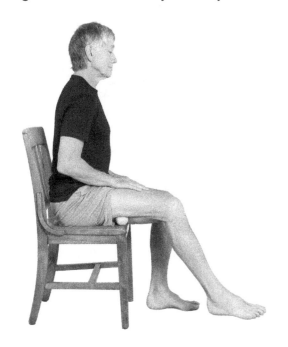

Switch sides.

Floor Variation: Sit on the floor with one or both legs extended. To make rolling easier, support yourself with your hands or with a bent leg to lift your bottom off the floor.

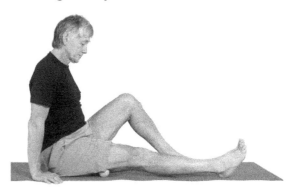

Double-Leg Stretch

Target: hamstrings, lower back

1. Sit on a mat with both legs straight out in front of you and your toes pointing up. Loop a strap around your feet and hold an end of the strap in each hand.

2. Gently pull yourself forward, keeping your back straight while you reach as far forward as is comfortable. Hold for as long as is comfortable, feeling the stretch in your lower back and the backs of your legs. Focus on keeping the legs straight.

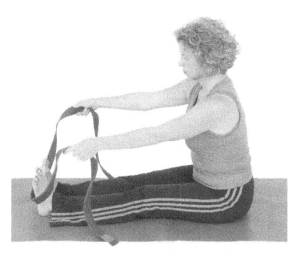

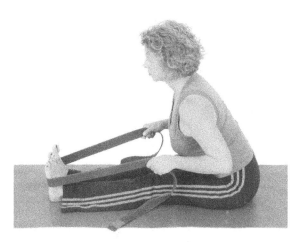

Variation: If you don't have a strap, you can gently press your thighs to the floor, your palms down on your thighs. If you have a partner, have him/her gently push you forward.

Advanced Variation: Interlace your fingers and reach forward, keeping your arms parallel to the floor.

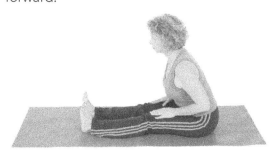

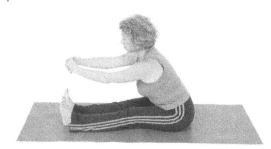

Standing Quad Stretch

Target: quadriceps

CAUTION: Avoid this exercise if you have poor balance. Stop if you notice undue compression in your knee or experience any lower back discomfort. If you feel a cramp coming on, stretch your hamstrings.

1. Stand with proper posture facing a chair. Loop a strap around your right ankle and bring your right heel toward your bottom. Keep both knees as close together as possible.

2. Gently pull your heel closer to your bottom, using the back of a chair for balance if necessary. Hold this stretch for a comfortable moment.

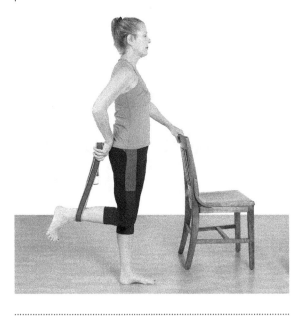

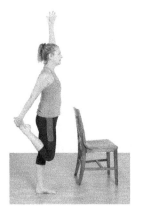

Switch sides and repeat.

Intermediate Variation: Try this without the strap by grabbing your foot with your hand.

Advanced Variation: Try this without the strap and the chair, raising your free arm toward the ceiling.

Side Quad Stretch

Target: quadriceps

CAUTION: Stop if you notice undue compression in your knee or experience any lower back discomfort. If you feel a cramp coming on, stretch your hamstrings.

1. Lie on the right side of your body on a mat. Keep your body in proper alignment: your left hip should be stacked on top of your right hip, your left knee on top of your right, your left shoulder on top of your right. Extend your bottom arm for balance. Loop a strap around your left ankle.

Advanced Variation: You can try this without the strap by grasping the top of your foot.

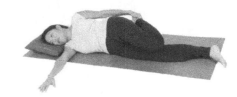

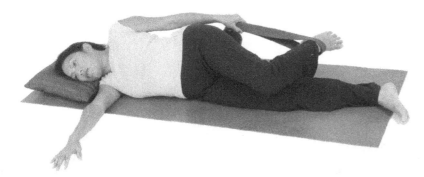

2. Gently bring the foot back, pulling your heel toward your bottom. Hold this stretch for a comfortable moment.

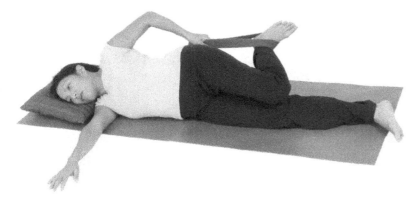

Switch sides and repeat.

Prone Quad Stretch

Target: quadriceps

1. Lie facedown on the mat with your legs straight.

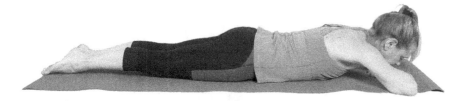

2. Bend your right leg toward your bottom and hold. If you feel a cramp coming on, stretch your hamstrings.

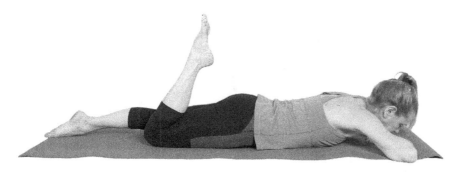

Perform with left leg.

Kneeling Quad Stretch

Target: quadriceps

CAUTION: Avoid this move if you have knee problems. You may want to kneel on a pad or mat to protect your knees.

1. Kneel in front of a chair. Place a pillow between your heels and your bottom, and place your hands on the chair.

2. Keeping both hands on the chair, slowly allow your bottom to drop toward your heels. Stop when you feel tension. Hold this stretch for a comfortable moment.

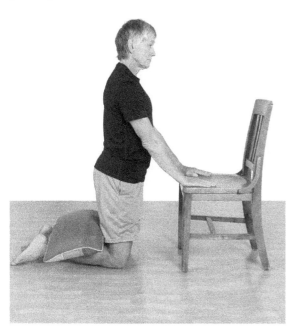

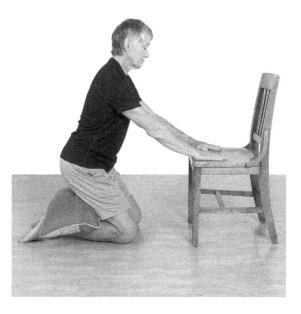

Variation: To increase the intensity of the stretch, use a flatter pillow, or eliminate the pillow altogether.

Quad Massage

Target: quadriceps

CAUTION: Avoid arching your lower back too much.

1. Lie facedown with your arms placed in a comfortable position to provide support. Place 1 or 2 small, firm balls (in a sock) under your thigh and just above your kneecap.

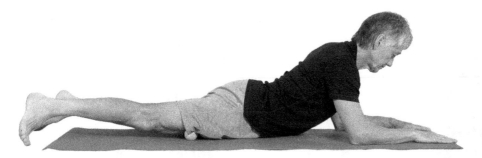

2. Roll the ball around under your thigh, controlling the pressure by shifting your weight. Use your intuition to guide you on how hard to press and where/how long to roll. Breathe slowly and fully.

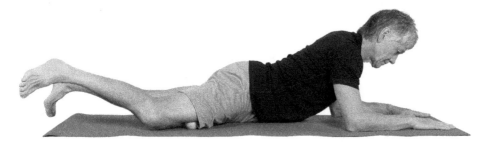

Switch sides.

Pretzel

Target: iliotibial band

1. Sit at the edge of a stable chair. Cross your left knee over your right.

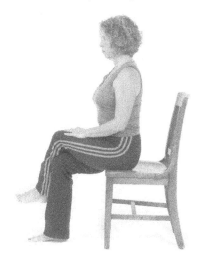

2. Reach both hands around the top of your left knee. Gently twist to the left while pulling the knee toward the midline of your body. Hold this stretch for a comfortable moment.

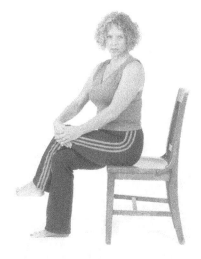

Switch sides and repeat.

Advanced Variation: This exercise can also be done sitting on the floor with your legs straight out in front of you. Bend your left knee and place your left foot on the outside of your right leg, as close to the right knee as possible. Then gently twist to the left as you look right.

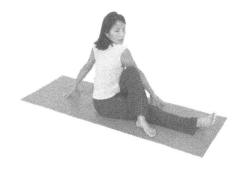

Outer Thigh Stretch

Target: iliotibial band

CAUTION: If you've been advised by your doctor or therapist not to cross your legs, do not do this exercise.

1. Stand with proper posture next to a chair on your left side. Cross your right leg in front of your left leg.

2. Raise your right arm up overhead and lean to the left, gently pressing your right hip outward to the right. Use the chair for balance. Hold this stretch for a comfortable moment.

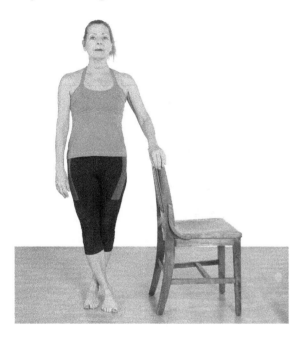

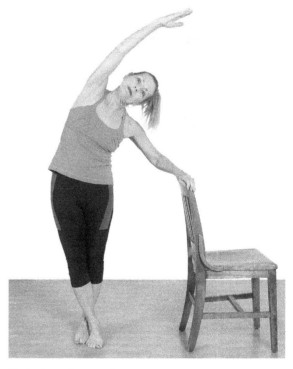

Switch sides and repeat.

Variation: If your shoulders are tight, just place your hand on your hips.

Advanced Variation: If balance is not an issue, try this without the chair.

Rear Calf Stretch

Target: calf

1. Stand behind a chair, placing both hands on the back of the chair. Keeping the heel down, slide your right leg as far back as you can.

2. Bend your left knee until the desired stretch is felt in the calf area. Hold this stretch for a comfortable moment.

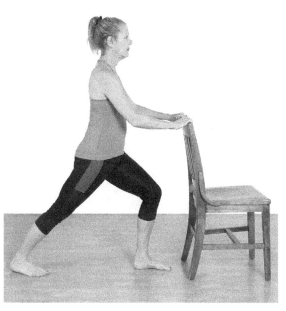

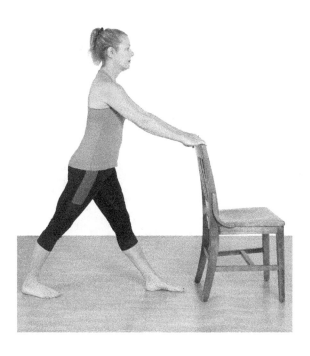

Switch sides and repeat.

Rear Calf Stretch with Strap

Target: calf

1. Stand with proper posture, holding a strap in your left hand. Step your left foot forward and loop the strap around the ball of the foot.

2. Keeping your heel on the floor, gently pull your toes up until you feel the desired stretch in your calf. Hold for a comfortable moment.

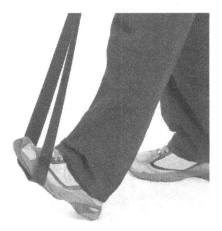

Switch sides and repeat.

Drop-Off Stretch

Target: calf

CAUTION: Only do this exercise if you're fairly flexible. Do not force anything, do not do this move if you have a history of Achilles' heel injury, and do not do this stretch if you're unsure of your balance.

1. Stand behind a chair, using the back for support. Place your right foot on a block.

2. Gently and slowly lower your right heel toward the floor until the desired stretch is felt in the calf area. Hold this stretch for a comfortable moment, using the chair for balance if necessary.

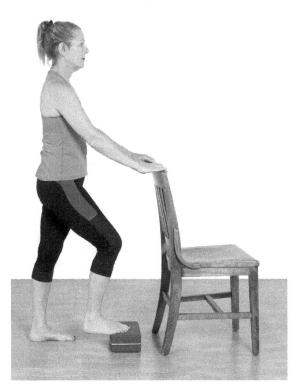

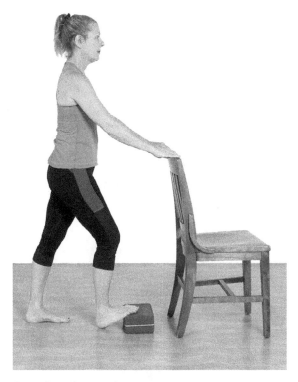

Switch sides and repeat.

Gas Pedal

Target: ankle

CAUTION: Do not force your toes in either direction. Be aware that your calf may cramp when extending your toes. Be careful not to tip the chair over.

1. Sit at the edge of a stable chair. Extend your left leg straight out in front of you and lift it off the ground.

2. Point your toes up and hold for several seconds.

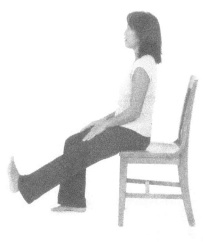

3. Extend your toes away from you and hold for several seconds.

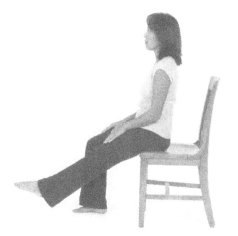

Resistance Band Variation: Wrap a resistance band around the ball of your foot once to keep it in place. Then perform the exercise.

Repeat a comfortable number of times then switch sides.

Heel Raise/Heel Drop

Target: ankle

1. Sit at the edge of a stable chair and place a block under the balls of your feet.

2. Keeping the balls of your feet on the block, raise your heels and hold the stretch for several seconds.

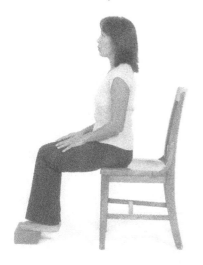

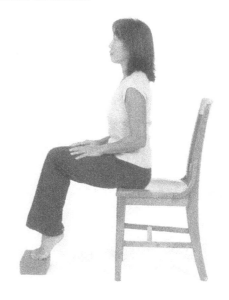

3. Drop your heels toward the floor and hold the stretch for several seconds.

Repeat a comfortable number of times.

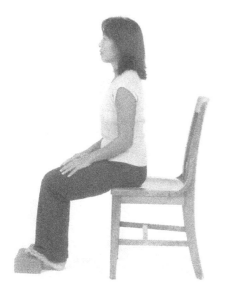

Ankle Circle

Target: ankle

1. Sit at the edge of a stable chair. Extend your left leg straight out in front of you and lift it off the ground.

2. Keeping your leg stationary (using your hands for support, if necessary), point your toes and draw several circles with your foot in both directions.

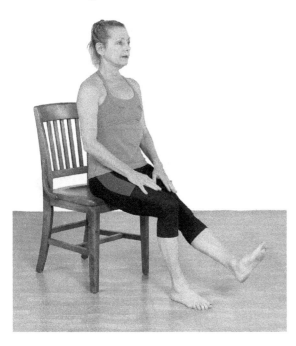

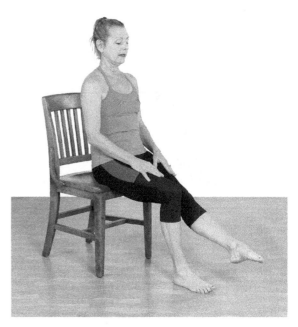

Switch sides and repeat.

Ankle Writing Variation: Point your toes and write your address and phone number with your foot. Switch sides and repeat.

Self ROM

Target: ankle

The Position: Sit at the edge of a stable chair. Cross your right ankle on top of your left knee and gently grasp your right foot with your left hand. Slowly use your hand to move your foot gently in comfortable circles as well as forward and backward.

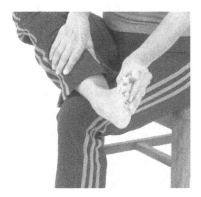 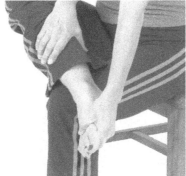 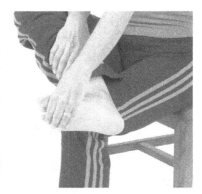

Switch sides and repeat.

Ankle Roller

Target: ankle

If you do not have a rolling pin, you can also use a frozen orange juice container (good for icing sore feet) or a can of soup.

1. Sit at the edge of a stable chair and place both feet on the floor, directly below your knees. Place a rolling pin under the arch of your right foot.

2. Slowly move your foot back and forth over the roller.

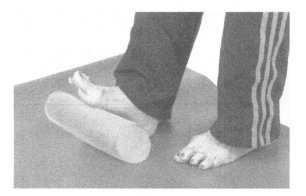

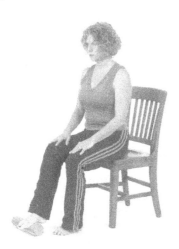

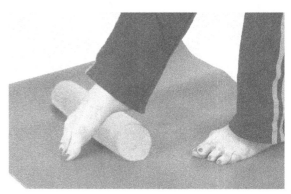

Switch sides and repeat.

Foot Massage

Target: foot

This can be done while standing or sitting.

The Position: If you have balance issues, standing by a wall or sitting are recommended. Place a small, firm ball under the ball of your foot. Roll the ball around under your entire foot and along the sides. Use your intuition to guide you on how hard to press and where/how long to roll. Breathe slowly and fully.

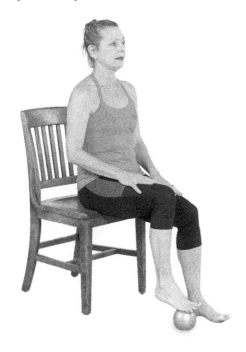

Switch sides.

Mad Cat

Target: total body

1. Rest on your hands and knees with your hands beneath your shoulders and knees beneath your hips.

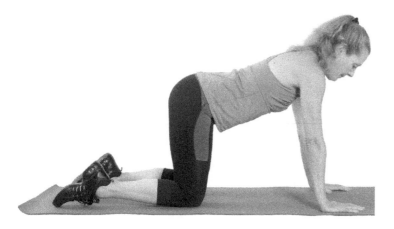

2. Draw your belly button in, causing your back to round. Inhale deeply.

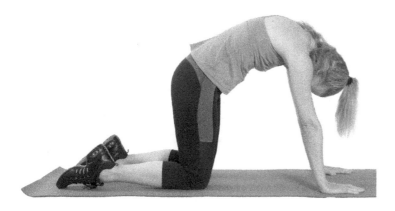

Now exhale and slowly relax your body to the starting position.

Repeat as desired.

Long Body Stretch

Target: total body

For this stretch, try listening to some relaxing music.

The Position: Lie on a mat, with your head on a pillow if needed. Focus on breathing slowly in and out through your nose. Reach your arms as far back as is comfortable. Lengthen your legs as far as is possible. Try to make your body as long as possible while breathing in a comfortable fashion. Remember to focus on your breath.

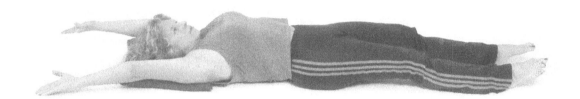

Index

Other Karl Knopf Books

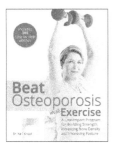

Beat Osteoporosis with Exercise
$15.95, 144pp
ISBN 978-1-61243-555-8
Beat Osteoporosis with Exercise provides the exercise and workout schedules that guarantee anyone, regardless of fitness level, can build strong bones.

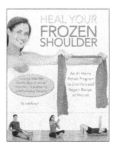

Heal Your Frozen Shoulder
$16.95, 144pp
ISBN 978-1-61243-643-2
With more than 50 step-by-step exercises, *Heal Your Frozen Shoulder* guarantees that anyone, regardless of fitness level, can recover from and prevent further shoulder pain.

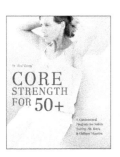

Core Strength for 50+
$15.95, 128pp
ISBN 978-1-61243-101-7
A fully illustrated guide to strengthening every aspect of the core muscles, tailored to the unique needs of aging adults.

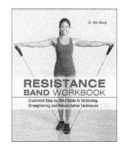

Resistance Band Workbook
$15.95, 120pp
ISBN 978-1-61243-171-0
The resistance band improves core strength, increases flexibility, tones muscles, releases tension, and rehabilitates injuries—all at home.

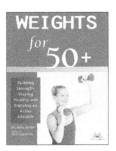

Weights for 50+
$15.95, 128pp
ISBN 978-1-56975-511-2
A fully illustrated program for the proper use of small "free weights" to maintain fitness and improve long-term health.

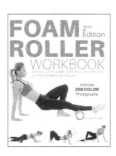

Foam Roller Workbook
2nd edition
$15.95, 112pp
ISBN 978-1-56975-925-7
Master the foam roller's versatility with this full-color, step-by-step guide to end pain, regain range of motion, and prevent injury using the foam roller.

To order these books call 800-377-2542 or 510-601-8301, fax 510-601-8307, e-mail ulysses@ulyssespress.com, or write to Ulysses Press, P.O. Box 3440, Berkeley, CA 94703. All retail orders are shipped free of charge. California residents must include sales tax. Allow two to three weeks for delivery.

Acknowledgments

Special thanks go to Casie Vogel for her vision and for making this book happen. Sincere appreciation goes to Claire Chun and her editing team, Lily Chou, Shayna Keyles, and Renee Rutledge, for their attention to detail. Another thought of appreciation goes to our models, Vivian Gunderson, Jack Holleman, Michael O'Meara, Phyllis Ritchie, and Toni Silver, for their patience and efforts. Lastly, my appreciation goes to Anja Ulfeldt of Rapt Productions and Robert Holmes for capturing the essence of the stretch.

About the Author

Dr. Karl Knopf (or Dr. Karl, as his students called him) was the director of the fitness therapy program at Foothill College for almost 40 years. During his tenure, he received several awards for teaching excellence. He retired in 2013. During his 45-plus years as a health and fitness professional, he worked in almost every aspect of the industry, including as a personal trainer (before the term was named), therapist at a VA hospital, and advisor to the State of California, as well as to several National Institutes of Health grants.

Dr. Karl has been a frequent speaker at national conferences and regional hospitals, and has appeared on public television's *Sit and Be Fit* show, as well as on their radio program. Over the years, Dr. Knopf has been interviewed for many print media publications, including the *Los Angeles Times* and *San Jose Mercury News*, and was featured in the *Wall Street Journal* on issues pertaining to senior fitness, exercise, and the disabled. He still authors articles and is still sought after for interviews. His Ulysses Press books (*Make the Pool Your Gym*, *Weights for 50+*, and *Core Strength for 50+*) are promoted in Tufts University health newsletters.

Currently, Dr. Knopf is the director of fitness therapy and senior fitness for the International Sports Science Association (ISSA) and is on the executive board of *Sit and Be Fit*. As a person who's over 65 years old, Dr. Knopf walks the talk. He still lifts weights, bikes, and swims daily while living with a chronic back and pain condition for over 30 years. He truly understands the importance of a daily stretch and being active to avoid surgery and over-reliance on pain medications. Dr. Karl firmly believes that what you do today determines how healthy and functional your tomorrow will be. His motto is "We may not be here for a long time, but grow well, not old!" Enjoy!